DE CONDITIONING *and* RE CONDITIONING

Earth Space Institute Book Series
Editor in Chief: Dr. Peter Kleber, Chairman, Earth Space Institute

The Earth Space Institute Book Series covers different aspects of the future of space. These books aim to show how space has become a new tool in further developments for the benefit of mankind. In this context, space can now be considered as part of the human experience. Each volume in the series will be devoted to selected topics in engineering, legal and financial issues, and space-based sciences (extraterrestrial, earth observation, life sciences, materials science) intended for students, researchers and space professionals. The series will also feature historical and general overviews of interest to the public.

DE CONDITIONING
and
RE CONDITIONING

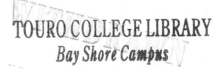

Edited by
John E. Greenleaf, Ph.D.

Research Physiologist (retired)
NASA Ames Research Center
Palo Alto, California

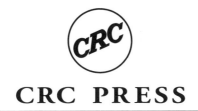

CRC PRESS

Boca Raton   London   New York   Washington, D.C.

BS

Library of Congress Cataloging-in-Publication Data

Deconditioning and reconditioning / edited by John E. Greenleaf
  p. cm. — (Earth Space Institute book series)
  Includes bibliographical references and index.
  ISBN 0-415-30650-7 (alk. paper)
  1. Hypokinesia—Physiological aspects. 2. Exercise therapy. I. Greenleaf, J. E. (John
Edward), 1932- II. Earth Space Institute book series on public and private sector interest
in space.

QP310.5.D43 2004
612′.04—dc22   2003067459

Visit the CRC Press Web site at www.crcpress.com

© 2004 by CRC Press LLC

No claim to original U.S. Government works
International Standard Book Number 0-415-30650-7
Library of Congress Card Number 2003067459
Printed in the United States of America 1 2 3 4 5 6 7 8 9 0
Printed on acid-free paper

10/11/06

Editor

John E. Greenleaf, Ph.D., a retired research physiologist at the NASA Ames Research Center near Palo Alto, California, is an adjunct professor in the Department of Human Performance at San Jose State University. Dr. Greenleaf earned his Ph.D. in human environmental physiology at the University of Illinois at Urbana–Champaign in 1963 and completed 1 year of post-doctoral research at the Karolinska Institute in Stockholm, Sweden in 1967. He has held graduate faculty and adjunct professor positions at San Francisco State University; University of Occupational and Environmental Health School of Medicine, Kitakyushu, Japan; University of Northern Colorado–Greely; University of California–Davis; and the Kyoto Prefectural University of Medicine.

Dr. Greenleaf is an internationally recognized scholar who has presented and published about 400 research abstracts, papers, book chapters, and review articles in the scientific literature. He is a member or emeritus member of Sigma Xi, the American Physiological Society, the Aerospace Medical Association (fellow), the American College of Sports Medicine (fellow), and the American Institute of Aeronautics and Astronautics (associate fellow). He is listed in *Who's Who in America*, and received distinguished alumni awards from New Mexico Highlands University and the University of Illinois, Department of Molecular and Integrative Physiology.

Acknowledgments

The authors thank very sincerely the extra effort provided by Charlotte Barton and Dani Thompson at NASA, Ames Research Center for administrative and editorial support, Lloyd Popish for editorial support, Nancy Mandella-Leone at Mandella Talent Annex for word processing of the book, James Donald at Boomerang Design Group for the preparation of figures, and David Faust for the cover design.

Introduction

Look at a patient lying long in bed. What a
pathetic picture he makes! The blood clotting
in his veins, the lime draining from his bones,
the scybala stacking up in his colon, the flesh
rotting from his seat, the urine leaking from his
distended bladder, and the spirit evaporating
from his soul.

R. A. J. Asher

Deconditioning is an integrated physiological response of the body to a reduction in metabolic rate; that is, to a reduction in energy use or in exercise level. While it may involve assumption of a horizontal body position, it certainly perturbs bodily homeostasis—at least temporarily. The reduction in physical activity that causes deconditioning is often associated with an increase in the time spent, for whatever reason, in a sitting or horizontal position. As a result, orthostatic factors may also contribute to the deconditioning mechanism.

The word *decondition* may be defined as "1: to cause extinction of (a conditioned response) 2: to cause to lose physical fitness" (*Webster's Collegiate Dictionary*, 105th ed., s.v. "decondition"). This definition implies that psychological/emotional factors may accompany physical deconditioning, and it is this interpretation of the word that is used throughout this volume.

It is apparent that deconditioning plays a major role in the mechanism of the general adaptive (homeostatic) response that is initiated by exposure to prolonged bed rest (BR). And the total homeostatic response to BR involves more than deconditioning per se. For example, it has been shown that the restoration of plasma volume and maximal work capacity after 4 weeks of BR-deconditioning left other bodily functions (submaximal exercise oxygen uptake and cardiac output, leg proprioception and posterior leg muscle thickness and volume, head-up tilt tolerance, and sleep quality) functioning at decreased levels. The precise effect of deconditioning on BR-homeostasis is difficult to determine, because the fundamental interactive neuro-endocrine-immune control networks that facilitate conditioning and deconditioning also act to maintain basic whole-body homeostasis. For example, is the mechanism of BR-induced deconditioning independent of the mechanism that provokes concomitant orthostatic intolerance, that is, fainting?

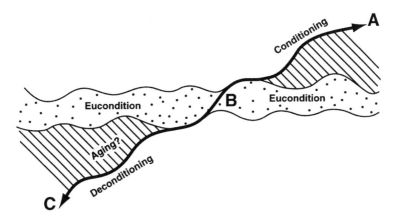

Assumption of the recumbent body position for prolonged periods of time results in a new adaptive-homeostatic state. This state occurs in response to the mutually interactive effects of the change in bodily position (hydrostatic pressure), to the virtual elimination of longitudinal pressure on the bones, to the increased confinement with possible reduction in total daily energy (exercise) expenditure, to the reorientation of stimuli within the vestibular organs, and (often) to altered socio-psychological conditions.

The conditioned and deconditioned states of the body are part of a continuum that includes the eucondition (see Figure), which is representative of the physical fitness range in which most people function in their daily lives. Exercise training can move the fitness level from B to A, whereas deconditioning (aging?) can move it from B to C. Many factors associated with various body positions (horizontal, sitting, standing) and degrees of immobilization (limb-casted, whole-body casted) contribute to deconditioning, and they must be considered when data from different studies are compared.

Partial deconditioning. In ambulatory subjects with either free movement in all planes, or with part of the body immobilized but with otherwise free movement in all spatial planes, the fitness shift is from A (conditioning) area to B (eucondition) area in the figure. If there is BR, immersion, or ambulatory confinement; and if (1) the whole body is free to move but only in the horizontal plane; or (2) if part of the body is immobilized with free movement only in the horizontal plane; or (3) if the whole body is immobilized (casted) with no movement in any plane, then the fitness shift is from B (eucondition) to C (deconditioning; aging) in the figure.

Maximal deconditioning. If there is BR, immersion, or ambulatory confinement the fitness shift is from A (conditioning) to C (deconditioning; aging) in the figure.

The exercise-training (reconditioning) syndrome affects total body homeostasis by facilitating increases in work capacity and endurance, whereas deconditioning decreases physical performance. There are many interrelated factors that influence the control parameters that seek to maintain the adaptive conditioning–deconditioning syndrome. These control parameters can be better elucidated by subjecting otherwise healthy ambulatory people to various stresses such as exercise training and prolonged spaceflight, bed rest, water immersion, hyperbaria, and isolation and confinement. Changes in control parameters will be manifested in muscle function, orthostatic tolerance, cardiorespiratory responses, musculo-skeletal systems, free-radical processes, and body thermoregulation with overarching effects on the subject's psycho-sociological states.

A discussion of these factors and the control parameters constitutes the substance of this volume. Special emphasis is placed on delineating practical applications of the findings that will be of special interest to physicians, nurses, and other health-care workers.

John E. Greenleaf

Contents

CHAPTER 1

Psycho-Sociological Aspects of Confinement Deconditioning

Gro M. Sandal[1], Ragnar Værnes[2], and Holger Ursin[3]

[1]*Department of Psychosocial Science, University of Bergen, Bergen, Norway*
[2]*Norwegian Underwater Technology Center, Bergen, Norway*
[3]*Department of Biological and Medical Psychology,
University of Bergen, Bergen, Norway*

> It is a man's own fault, it is from want of use,
> if his mind grows torpid in old age.
>
> *Samuel Johnson*

INTRODUCTION

Deconditioning, the physiological response to reduced activity, involves psychological changes that may contribute to further inactivity by means of positive feedback; the resulting changes in the musculoskeletal system may be an important cause of the frequent complaints and sickness certifications concerning muscle pain (Ursin et al.,1993). This restricted activity is related to motivational factors and to an active choice of lifestyle. However, we will only deal with deconditioning as it occurs under circumstances in which normal activity is restricted because of environmental factors. Included will be data from isolation studies conducted as simulations of prolonged space journeys, data from other long-term isolation studies, and data from submarine expeditions, treks to polar regions, and diving experiments. The emphasis here will be on psychological factors, including psychophysiological, psychoendocrine, and psychoimmune parameters that affect the performance of individuals and groups; on what changes occur, and on how to identify and counteract them. To some extent proper selection, training, and other organization of individuals may prevent these adverse changes. Recommendations will be made regarding the composition and training of groups that have to live together in isolation for long periods and perform to high standards under stressful conditions.

Weightlessness in space does not induce unique psychological problems except for the novelty and inconveniences, and the necessity of being able to cope with them. The real psychological challenges that are peculiar to space are the isolation and the hazardous environment, living with the same few people for prolonged periods, and the potential stress of escape and evacuation. This physical deconditioning does not induce serious psychological challenges, at least during the mission (Ursin et al., 1993). However, serious psychological changes may indeed affect all other physiological parameters through the motivation for adaptation and prevention.

Suedfeld and colleagues refer to these situations as "capsule environments" and define isolated, confined environments (ICE) as a subset of extreme, unusual environments (EUE) (Suedfeld, 1987; Suedfeld and Steel, 2000). The external environmental and restricting factors make the internal environment important, and the psychological and social environments become even more important because there is no escape from the group. The dynamics of the group influence each individual, and each individual influences the group; this well-being, performance, and in some cases survival of the crew members depend on the coherence, effectiveness, and interactions between them.

Thus, the principal purpose of this chapter is to discuss the psychological changes that occur when humans live in isolated environments in which physical activity is limited and deconditioning is induced. We will also discuss the reciprocal effects; that is, those of reconditioning. To what extent do the psychological changes contribute to the deconditioning state, and to what extent does deconditioning affect psychological factors? Finally, we will describe briefly how potentially disastrous effects may be counteracted by subject selection procedures, group composition, training, and other preventive actions undertaken before, during and after the isolation.

PSYCHOLOGICAL REACTIONS TO CONFINEMENT

Psychological factors are assumed to be a primary limiting condition for long-duration spaceflights (Collet et al., 1991). Personnel working in space or in other ICE may be exposed to unacceptably high levels of stress that might interfere with their performance of assigned duties, with their health, and even with mission success. Documented psychological and psychophysiological responses to spaceflights and other ICE include transient disorientation and spatial illusion, mild cognitive impairment, interpersonal tension, and degradation of performance (Rivolier, 1997).

Interpersonal issues will become increasingly important as space missions become longer and crews become more heterogeneous as to experience, professional background, and assigned duties (Helmreich, 1983). Data from aircrews have shown that tension results in inefficient communication that may cause errors and interfere with safety (Foushee and Manos, 1981). Interpersonal reactions that have often occurred include (1) displacement of aggression to outside personnel; (2) "scapegoating" of crew members deviating from the rest of the group; (3) formation of subgroups along national or vocational lines; (4) unstable command structure; and (5) tension and conflicts between crew members leading to territorial behavior and withdrawal from group interaction.

Resistance and mistrust of outsiders, often referred to as the "us versus them" phenomenon, is one mechanism that unites isolated groups (Nicholas and Foushee, 1990). However, such intergroup tension might inhibit communication and interfere with the capacity of the group to accurately receive and process information from outside personnel, thereby resulting in errors of judgment and in performance decrements. How to control this phenomenon should therefore be addressed in the preparation for such missions. In the context of prolonged spaceflight, this problem also suggests the potential danger of relying too heavily on Earth-based command and support mechanisms (Nicholas and Foushee, 1990).

It is important to understand the critical periods that occur during crew performance and adaptation. It has been assumed that there are long-term costs of adapting to chronic stressors associated with isolated, operational environments. Length of stay in long-term, confined, and isolated environments correlates positively with increased blood pressure and plasma catecholamine concentrations, and with negative moods (Cohen et al., 1986). One important determinant of psychological reactions is knowledge or expectancy of the end of the situation (Gushin et al., 1993). Rohrer (1961) described three broad stages of psychological reactions to prolonged stays in Antarctic groups: (1) heightened anxiety, (2) settling down to routine marked by depression, and (3) anticipation of termination of the situation marked by emotional outbursts, aggressiveness, and rowdy behavior. An important aspect of a stage-model of adaptation is that these reactions are assumed to occur in the same relative phases of the isolation, independent of the actual duration and characteristics of the environments. The experimental designs of many studies have been directed toward confirming the occurrence of such critical phases. During simulation studies in hyperbaric chambers, interpersonal tension increased from the middle toward the end of the isolation (Sandal et al., 1995; Sandal, 2001). Other data suggest that psychological reactions in different environments change differently. Both Palinkas et al. (1998) and Sandal (2001) found that groups in different Antarctic environments exhibited different time patterns of psychological reactions. In a previous study we compared space simulation data with data collected during polar crossings (Sandal et al., 1996). Under the former conditions, personal coping increased gradually over time which was attributed to the relatively safe and predictable conditions in the chambers. Members in polar crossing studies displayed a marked reduction in anxiety and aggression from the second to the third quarter of their journey, whereas homesickness increased noticeably over the course of the expedition.

The ability to predict psychological and interpersonal problems would enable both space crew members and outside personnel to intervene before those problems degraded health or operational situations. If participants expect undesirable incidents, then problems might be handled with greater tact because they would not be personalized. Such knowledge might ameliorate untoward consequences such that habitat design, work tasks, and schedules might be planned to minimize social and psychological problems. Different strategies for lighting schedules, celebrations, or distracting tasks might also reduce the negative effects of foreseen crises (Harrison et al., 1990). In general, the need for privacy seems to increase with the duration of isolation and this need should be addressed in planning living compartments and scheduling free and leisure time for long-duration missions (Harrison et al., 1990).

PERSONNEL SELECTION

A critical component of any personnel selection procedure is to identify the attributes required to perform the job successfully. The objective of selection strategies is twofold: to eliminate unfit applicants, and to select from otherwise qualified candidates those who will perform optimally. An important distinction is therefore made between "selecting out" and "selecting in" criteria. Candidates need to be selected-out for medical and psychiatric disorders in an early phase of the process. The psychological selected-in criteria can be divided into two categories: operational aptitudes, and personality factors. In relation to operational aptitudes, it is important that candidates show above average performance for cognitive and psychomotor capabilities in logical reasoning, mental arithmetic, visual and auditory memory function, attention, perception, spatial comprehension, and psychomotor coordi-nation. Selection criteria for astronauts related to personality have included motiv-ation, social capabilities, stress coping, and work orientation (Santy, 1994). In the following sections we will focus on how these factors might be facilitated.

Personality

Personality is often defined as stable, deep-seated dispositions to respond in particu-lar ways, and is reflected in relatively stable behavior over time that is consistent across situations. To the extent that desired behavior during confinement is related to stable traits, training is unlikely to produce desired changes. In fact, data from studies of the effects of cockpit resource management (CRM) training indicated that personality dispositions represented important limitations for the ability of military pilots to benefit from training (Chidester et al., 1991). An important implication of these findings is that approaches to ensure optimal crew performance need to balance selection and training strategies.

   Individuals who cope and perform successfully under stressful conditions seem to have traits in common that differentiate them from those who do not; that is, they show lower anxiety and less fear when in dangerous situations, have high achieve-ment motivation (Foushee, 1981), have high need for external change, and thrive on adventure and mastering difficult tasks (Rachman, 1991). These personality charac-teristics have been described as positive response outcome expectancies, typical of individuals who learn to cope and master stressful and difficult tasks (Levine and Ursin, 1991). The individual expectations of personal control in the specific situation seem to determine the stress response, both at the psychological level and at the physiological level with activation of the autonomic, endocrine, and immune systems.

Defensive Strategies

An important factor in expectancy of control is use of defensive strategies. Defense is most likely to occur when no means of coping is available and when the level of fear is high (Lazarus et al., 1974). The central aspect of this concept is that the trait is linked to the perception of the threat by the subject. By using tests of defensive strategies; that is, in the selection process, there is a shift in emphasis from the level of anxiety aroused or the intensity of the threat to the various ways in which the subjects handle and perceive the challenging (threatening) situation. There is considerable evidence for this position from empirical studies based on the following experimental designs: longitudinal studies on serious near-miss and fatal accidents; relationship to performance impairment in the threatening situation; relationship to endocrine activation in threatening situations; and relationship to perceived health complaints and immune reactions.

For evaluating defensive strategies the Defense Mechanism Test (DMT) is often used (Kragh, 1960, 1962). The basic assumption of the test is that if anxiety-arousing stimuli are used, then individual differences in the perceptual process may give insight into aspects of individual strategies for coping with the stress. In one longitudinal study, Neuman (1978) analyzed the predictive value of the DMT among Swedish air force pilots over a 10-year period. Of 225 trainees, 136 passed basic training; of this group, 63 had high defense (HD) scores on the DMT and 73 had low defense (LD) scores on the DMT. Of the 63 HD subjects, 6 died in flight accidents while none in the LD group died in flight accidents. Furthermore, 15 of the 17 accidents with "total loss of aircraft" came from the HD group. Thus, those with higher defense scores appear to have performed poorly.

In performance research, Værnes (1982) and Værnes and Darragh (1982) studied how defensive reactions (measured by DMT) among deep sea divers related to more specific reduction in performance. Among the 44 divers tested at a depth of 60 m, there was a significant positive correlation ($r = 0.39$, $p < 0.02$) between reasoning impairment and high defense scores. Furthermore, when combining manifest anxiety (MA) and high scores on the reaction formation (RF) variable, of the 11 divers who had high MA and RF scores, 9 had impairment of reasoning that exceeded the group median score (20%); among the 11 divers who had low MA and RF scores, none showed a reduction in reasoning that placed it below the median. These results support the usefulness of the DMT when combined with anxiety tests for predicting poor performance in dangerous tasks.

Baade et al. (1978) published the first study in which DMT scores were correlated with psychobiological measures of activation (stress response). Forty-four parachute trainees were followed through their training period; factor analysis of multiple endocrine measures (cortisol, growth hormone, testosterone, prolactin, epinephrine, and norepinephrine) did not indicate the presence of a single activation factor. Rather, three factors emerged; cortisol, testosterone, and catecholamines. These endocrine factors related differently to psychological factors, suggesting that they reflected independent nervous and endocrine response systems regarding effects of psychological activation. The DMT scores correlated positively and significantly ($p < 0.005$)

with the cortisol factor and to not-accepted parachute jumps, again confirming that DMT data predicted poor performance in dangerous tasks.

The data mentioned above indicated that defensive strategies may be dangerous in situations in which survival depends on immediate and precise action. The defensive strategy may also affect health parameters on long-term moderately stressful situations. Increased experience in coping with stress together with interpersonal difficulties can lead to lower immunoglobulin levels, a long-term indicator of stress and health risk factors (McClelland et al., 1980; Reily, 1981; Ursin et al., 1984; Endresen et al., 1989; Værnes et al., 1988, 1991). Værnes et al. (1987) analyzed data from 23 submarine officers concerning relationships between personality factors and transitory/chronic health problems perceived during and after cruise missions. There was a higher frequency of perceived health problems among these subjects than with those in other respective occupations; the problems were mainly pain in the neck/shoulders (22% during the mission, 9% after the mission), stomach problems (48% versus 0%), headache (22% versus 4%), and general lethargy (61% versus 44%). Low immunoglobulin A (IgA) levels were correlated significantly ($r = 0.62$, $p < 0.02$) with health complaints during cruise missions and with high defense scores on the DMT.

Findings from a study of 45 North Sea saturation divers in a hyperbaric diving bell (Bergan et al., 1987) indicated significant negative correlations between immune levels and environmental factors: DMT scores correlated with both low IgG ($r = -0.44$, $p < 0.05$) and low complement component C3 ($r = -0.46$, $p < 0.05$). There were also several positive correlations between low immune levels and experience (number of days in saturation) indicating that long-term stress may lead to immune-related health problems. Divers with high DMT scores had significantly more sleep problems in the hyperbaric condition than those with low scores; those with a higher number of accidents had both high trait anxiety and high DMT scores that correlated highly ($r = 0.45$, $p < 0.05$) with the number of accidents within the diving bell.

Motivation

Motivation is the degree of interest and enthusiasm an individual exhibits for a given job or task. Generally, astronauts must have a high degree of mission-oriented motivation and a lesser degree of personal motivational factors (Santy, 1994). Competitive individuals who are driven by a desire to outperform others are likely to generate interpersonal stress and hostility, adversely affecting collaborative performance and further undermining the quality of the social environment which may already have been compromised by the stressful conditions. These considerations strengthen the postulate that astronauts should exhibit a strong willingness and desire to master challenging tasks *as a team*.

Interpersonal Capabilities

Lack of interpersonal sensitivity might interfere with performance on tasks that require interaction and cooperation with others in a restricted living area. This lack of sensitivity may be counteracted by proper composition of the group. For example, preference should be given to individuals who are caring and sensitive to the needs of other people but, at the same time, they must also be sufficiently task- and achievement-motivated to be able to cope and perform in isolated and confined situations (Chidester et al., 1991; McFadden et al., 1994; Sandal et al., 1995; Sandal et al., 1998, 1999). Interpersonal compatibility is determined, in part, by personality factors, for example, by levels of achievement-motivation, and individual dominance (Helmreich and Wilhelm, 1985). Also, similarities in values and attitudes might determine whether people get along at an interpersonal level. Data from studies conducted in different isolated and confined space, such as during Antarctic expeditions, in submarines and in hyperbaric chambers, have demonstrated that subjects who are both highly achievement-motivated and interpersonally sensitive show superior performance. This personality profile has been referred to as the "Right Stuff" in stressful team environments to describe optimal psychological attributes in aerospace situations (Wolfe, 1979; King and Flynn, 1996). Poorer performance has been linked to personality profiles typified by a hostile, competitive, interpersonal orientation ("Wrong Stuff"), and to low achievement-motivation combined with passive-aggressive characteristics ("No Stuff"). These personality profiles have been evaluated and utilized in the selection of astronauts (Maki et al., 1991; McFadden et al., 1994).

COUNTERMEASURES FOR ALLEVIATING PSYCHOLOGICAL PROBLEMS IN ESTABLISHED CREWS

The psychological training of people who are to be exposed to occupational confinement requires that individual aptitudes, attitudes, and skills be improved to prepare them to meet mission demands (Manzey et al., 1995) with focus on both the individual's ability to cope and perform, as well as on efficient coordination and cooperation within the group setting. For example, support techniques and interventions during spaceflights might be designed to reduce or prevent psychological and interpersonal problems. To detect such problems, space mission crews have been evaluated by communication with mission control (Gushin et al., 1997; Kanas, 1991) by means of speech analysis which included intonational and time characteristics (duration of communication sessions, talking speed, and silences) and themes discussed. Analyses of communication sessions have provided empirical evidence for the appearance of several factors that are assumed to reflect the psychological climate within the crew and that affect the interaction between them and outside personnel. Such factors have included psychological closing, a tendency of crew members to avoid sharing their feelings with others, and information filtration in crew communication (Gushin et al., 1996).

For personnel working under hazardous conditions, attention should be paid to indicators of wakefulness and awareness, for example, overt behavior, electroencephalographic recordings, and neuropsychological tests. Ursin et al. (1991) have emphasized the importance of registering deviations and indications of a breakdown in group organization and coherence, because serious psychological difficulties may necessitate the evacuation of personnel or termination of the project.

To distinguish significant psychological deviations from the norm requires previously obtained reference data for each individual that record normal variations in any given behavioral parameter (Hockey, 1992). There is an inherent difficulty when monitoring performance in that the error thresholds must be operationally meaningful. Is the performance "good enough", even if there is a variance from baseline? The more "central" responses (mood, memory, attention) are best measured by specially designed tasks that reflect changes in working memory and control processing, as opposed to automatic processing. There seems to be limited value in using standard measurements of reaction time (e.g., Sternberg test); they are not sensitive to changes in capacity or mental state, but reflect mainly stable differences between individuals. Any change in such capabilities may reflect a general loss of motivation (Hockey, 1992).

Reliable questionnaires, which have been tested for reliability, validity, and acceptance, are available for use in evaluating mood, motivation, cognitive factors, and subjective health complaints (Ursin et al., 1991). The transfer of information directly to the individual in a digested, positive, and understandable form is a primary element in all applications of contemporary psychological principles. Also, corrective action should be instigated by the affected person, if possible. Therefore, the corrective information should be fed back clearly to the individual as soon as possible. An essential part of the social group observation system's self-evaluation of each group member's performance and function is that the self-evaluations may be compared with those made by the other group members.

CONCLUSIONS

From experience with those in confined environments, it seems reasonable to conclude that psychological countermeasures are key factors for use in any long-duration confinement program. They are most effective when they are specifically designed for the demands of a given mission and when they address not only the crew or the test subjects, but also their families, key external personnel, and those conducting the test. Efficient countermeasures include appropriate selection, composition, training, and support of the test participants.

REFERENCES

Baade, E., Halse, K., Stenhammer, P. E., Ellertsen, B., Johnsen, T. B., and Vollmer, F. (1978) Psychological Tests. In *Psychobiology of Stress: A Study of Coping Men*, edited by H. Ursin, E. Baade, and S. Levine, Academic Press: New York, pp. 125–160.
Bergan, T., Værnes, R. J., Ingebrigsten, P., Tønder, O., Aakvaag, A., and Ursin, H. (1987) Relationships between work environmental problems and health among Norwegian

divers in the North Sea. In *Diving and Hyperbaric Medicine*, edited by A. Marroni and G. Oriani, EUBS: Palermo, pp. 327–336.

Chidester, T. R., Helmreich, R. L., Gregorich, E. and Geis, C. E. (1991) Pilot personality and crew coordination: implications for training and selection. *Int. J. Aviat. Psychol.* **1**: 25–44.

Cohen, S., Evans, G. W., Stokels, D., and Krantz, D. (1986) *Stress and the Environment.* Putnam: New York.

Collet, J., Gharib, C. I., Kirsch, K., and Værnes, R. J. (1991) Scientific results from the ISEMSI experiment. *ESA Bull.* **17**: 483–487.

Endressen, I., Værnes, R. J., Ursin, H., and Tønder, O. (1989) Psychological stress factors and concentrations of immunoglobulins and complement components in Norwegian nurses. *Work Stress* **4**: 365–375.

Foushee, H. C. (1981) The role of communication, socio-psychology, and personality factors in the maintenance of crew coordination. *Aviat. Space Environ. Med.* **53**: 1062–1066.

Foushee, H. C., and Manos, K. L. (1981) Information transfer within the cockpit: problems in intracockpit communication. In *Information Transfer Problems in the Aviation System*, NASA TR-1875, edited by C. E. Billings and E. S. Cheaney.

Gushin, V. I., Kholin, S. F., and Ivanovsky, Y. R. (1993) Soviet psychophysiological investigations of simulated isolation. In *Advances in Space Biology and Medicine*, edited by S. Bonting, JAI Press, Inc: London, pp. 5–14.

Gushin, V. I., Kolintchenko, V. A., Efimov, V. A., Davies, C. (1996) Psychological evaluation and support during EXEMSI. In *Advances in Space Biology and Medicine*, edited by S. Bonting, JAI Press Inc.: London, pp. 283–296.

Gushin, V. I., Zaprisa, T. B., Kolintchenko, V. A., Efimov, A., Smirnova, T. M., Vinokhodova, A. G., and Kanas, N. (1997) Content analysis of the crew communication with external communicants under prolonged isolation. *Aviat. Space Environ. Med.* **12**: 1093–1098.

Harrison, A., Clearwater, Y. A., and McKay, C. P. (1990) The human experience in Antarctica: applications to life in space. *Behav. Sci.* **34**: 253–271.

Helmreich, R. L. (1983) Applying psychology in outer space: unfulfilled promises revisited. *Am. Psychol.* **38**: 445–450.

Helmreich, R. L., and Wilhelm, J. A. (1985) The undersea habitat as a space station analog: evaluation of research and training potential, NASA/University of Texas Report, pp. 85–87.

Hockey, G. R. J. (1992) Report of working group on maintenance of performance. In *Integrated Monitoring in Space*: *Space Psychology Days 2*, edited by A. W. H. Galliard, European Space Agency LTPO-SR92-01, Paris.

Kanas, N. (1991) Psychological support for cosmonauts. *Aviat. Space Environ. Med.* **63**: 353–355.

King, R. E., and Flynn, C. F. (1996) Defining and measuring the "right stuff" – neuropsychiatric flight screening. *Aviat. Space Environ. Med.* **66**: 951–956.

Kragh, U. (1960) The Defense Mechanism Test: a new method for diagnosis and personnel selection. *J. Appl. Psychol.* **44**: 303–309.

Kragh, U. (1962) Prediction of success of Danish attack divers by the Defense Mechanism Test (DMT). *Percept. Mot. Skills* **15**: 103–106.

Lazarus, R. S., Averill, J. R., and Opton, E. M. (1974) The psychology of coping: Issues of research and assessment. In *Coping and Adaptation*, edited by G. V. Coelho, D. A. Hamburg, and J. E. Adams. Basic Books: New York.

Levine, S., and Ursin, H. (1991) What is stress? In *Stress-Neurobiology and Neuroendocrinology*, edited by M. R. Brown, G. F. Koob, and C. Rivier, Marcel Dekker: New York.

Maki, P., Pettersen, R., Olff, M., Sandal, G., Warncke, M., and Ursin, H. (1991) Collection of normative data: Psychodynamics under stress. WP 640. In *Definition of Psychological Testing of Astronaut Candidates for Columbus Missions,* edited by K. M. Goeters and C. Fassbender, European Space Agency, 9730/90/NL/IW.

Manzey, D., Schiewe, A., and Fassbender, C. (1995) Psychological countermeasures for extended manned spaceflights. *Acta Astronautica* **35**: 339–361.

McClelland, D. C., Davidson, R. J., Floor, E., and Saron, C. (1980) Stresses power motivation, sympathetic activation, immune function and illness. *J. Hum. Stress* **6**: 6–15.

McFadden, T. J., Helmreich, R., Rose, R. M., and Fogg, L. F. (1994) Predicting astronauts effectiveness: a multivariant approach. *Aviat. Space Environ. Med.* **65**: 904–909.

Neuman, T. (1978) Dimensionering och validering av perceptgenesen for forsvarsmekanismer. En hierarkisk analys mot pilots stress beteende. FOA Report No. 55020-H6, Sweden.

Nicholas, J. M., and Foushee, H. C. (1990) Organization, selection, and training of crews for extended spaceflight: findings from analogs and implications. *J. Spacecraft* **27**: 451–456.

Palinkas, L. A., Johnson, J. C., Boster, A. S., and Houseal, M. (1998) Longitudinal studies of behavior and performance during a winter at the South Pole. *Aviat. Space Environ. Med.* **69**: 73–77.

Rachman, S. J. (1991) Psychological analyses of courageous performance in military personnel. Defense Technical Information Center; Alexandria, Rept. ARI-RN-91-86, VA.

Reily, V. (1981) Psychoneuroendocrine influences in immunocompetence and neoplasia. *Science* **212**: 1100–1109.

Rivolier, J. (1997) L'homme dans l'espace: Une approche psycho-écologique des vols habitués. Presses Universitaires de France: Paris.

Rohrer, J. (1961) Interpersonal relationships in isolated small groups. In *Psychological Aspects of Manned Spaceflight*, edited by B. Flaherty, Columbia University Press: New York.

Sandal, G. M. (2000) Coping in Antarctica: Is it possible to generalize across environments? *Aviat. Space Environ. Med.* **71:** (9, Suppl.) A37–43.

Sandal, G. M. (2001) Crew tension during a space station simulation. *Environ. Behav.* **33, 1:** 135–150.

Sandal, G. M., Bergan, T., Warncke, M., Værnes, R. J., and Ursin, H. (1996) Psychological reactions during polar expeditions and isolation in hyperbaric chambers. *Aviat. Space Environ. Med.* **67**: 227–234.

Sandal, G. M., Endresen, I., Værnes, R., and Ursin, H. (1999) Personality and coping strategies during submarine missions. *Mil. Psychol.* **11**: 381–403.

Sandal, G. M., Groenningsaeter, H., Eriksen, H. R., Gravraakmo, A., Birkeland, K., and Ursin, H. (1998) Personality and endocrine activation in military stress situations. *Mil. Psychol.* **10**: 45–61.

Sandal, G. M., Værnes, R., and Ursin, H. (1995) Interpersonal relations in space simulation studies. *Aviat. Space Environ. Med.* **66**: 617–624.

Santy, P. (1994) *Choosing the Right Stuff: the Psychological Selection of Astronauts and Cosmonauts*. Prager: London.

Suedfeld, P. (1987) Extreme and unusual environments. In *Handbook of Environmental Psychology*, Vol. 1, edited by D. Stokols and I. Altman, Wiley: New York, pp. 863–886.

Suedfeld, P., and Steel, G. D. (2000) The environmental psychology of capsule habitats. *Annu. Rev. Psychol.* **51**: 227–253.

Ursin, H., Endresen, I. M., Svebak, S., Tellnes, G., and Mykletun, R. (1993) Muscle pain and coping with working life in Norway: a review. *Work Stress* **7**: 247–258.

Ursin, H., Mykletun, R., Tønder, O., Værnes, R. J., Relling, G., Isaksen, E., and Murison, R. (1984) Psychological stress-factors and concentrations of immunoglobulins and complement components in humans. *Scand. Psychol.* **23**: 340–347.

Ursin, H., Værnes, R., Endresen, I. M., and Warncke, M. (1991) Physiological and psychological aspects of living in confined space under strenuous conditions. *Scott Polar Record, Polar Symposia* **1**: 39–42.

Værnes, R. J. (1982) The Defense Mechanism Test predicts inadequate performance under stress. *Scand. J. Physiol.* **23**: 37–43.

Værnes, R. J., and Darragh, A. (1982) Endocrine reactions and cognitive performance at 60 metres hyperbaric pressure: correlations with perceptual defense reactions. *Scand. J.*

Physiol. **23**: 193–199.

Værnes, R. J., Knardahl, S., Ursin, H., and Rømsing, J. (1988) Relations between environmental problems, psychology and health among shift-workers in the Norwegian process-industry. *Work Stress* **2**: 7–15.

Værnes, R. J., Myhre, G., Aas, H., Homnes, T., Hansen, I., and Tønder, O. (1991) Relationships between stress, psychological factors, health, and immune levels among military aviators. *Work Stress* **5**: 5–16.

Værnes, R. J., Warncke, M., Eidsvik, S., Aakvaag, A., Tønder, O., and Ursin, H. (1987) Relationships between perceived health and psychological factors among submarine personnel: endocrine and immunological effects. In *Diving and Hyperbaric Medicine*, edited by A. Marroni and G. Oriani, EUBS: Palermo, pp. 19–28.

Wolfe, T. (1979) *The Right Stuff.* Farrar, Straus and Giroux: New York.

CHAPTER 2

Effects of Deconditioning and Reconditioning on Aerobic Power

Victor A. Convertino

US Army Institute of Surgical Research, Fort Sam, Houston, Texas, USA

> Who, doomed to go in company with Pain,
> And Fear, and Bloodshed, miserable train!
> Turns his necessity to glorious gain;
> In face of these doth exercise a power …
>
> *William Wadsworth*

INTRODUCTION

Maximal oxygen uptake ($\dot{V}O_{2\,max}$), often referred to as aerobic capacity, is defined as the highest rate at which the whole body can utilize oxygen. $\dot{V}O_{2\,max}$ is generally regarded as the best single measurement of cardiorespiratory endurance and aerobic physical fitness. Since deconditioning can be defined as the loss of physical fitness, measurement of alterations in $\dot{V}O_{2\,max}$ during exposure to bed rest (BR) or spaceflight should provide an accurate assessment of the magnitude of the deconditioning process on the cardiovascular system.

The Fick equation expresses the relationship between the oxygen uptake ($\dot{V}O_2$, the amount of oxygen utilized by the total human body), A-$\dot{V}O_{2\,diff}$ [difference between the arterial and venous concentrations of oxygen resulting from the amount of oxygen extracted by the working muscles, and cardiac output (heart rate, HR, times stroke volume, SV)]: thus $\dot{V}O_2 = HR \times SV \times A\text{-}\dot{V}O_{2\,diff}$.

Therefore, identification and understanding of mechanisms that underlie alterations in $\dot{V}O_{2\,max}$ during the deconditioning process can be assessed by evaluating changes in factors that influence the control of heart rate, stroke volume, and oxygen delivery and utilization. Therefore, the purpose of this chapter is to critically review and integrate data to better understand the possible mechanistic adaptations that dictate the reduction in aerobic fitness in people confined to BR or who participate in spaceflight, and discuss possible approaches to the development of effective countermeasures to reverse the problem.

DECONDITIONING RESULTS FROM BED REST

Aerobic power or $\dot{V}O_{2\,max}$ is reduced by as much as 5 to 35% in subjects confined to BR (Table 2.1; Convertino, 1986, 1997; Greenleaf and Kozlowski, 1982a,b). The magnitude of its loss is dependent upon the duration of confinement; and the relative reduction (%Δ) in $\dot{V}O_{2\,max}$ with BR appears to be similar across gender and age groups (Convertino, 1986; Convertino et al., 1977, 1986a). However, there is a tendency for highly fit individuals who have greater $\dot{V}O_{2\,max}$ to demonstrate greater absolute and relative reduction in their aerobic power compared to more sedentary people (Convertino, 1986; Convertino et al., 1986a; Convertino, 1998; Saltin et al. 1968), although exceptions to this relationship have been reported due to differences in methods of measurement (Greenleaf and Kozlowski, 1982a,b). Therefore, duration of confinement and initial level of fitness appear to be determinants of the reduction in aerobic power induced by BR.

Mechanisms for maximal heart rate. After exposure to BR, the heart rate is elevated at the same oxygen requirement, including that at maximal physical effort (Convertino, 1983, 1986, 1987, 1997; Convertino et al., 1977, 1982a,b,c, 1986a; Deitrick et al., 1948; Georgiyevskiy et al., 1966; Kashihara et al., 1994; Stremel et al. 1976; Suzuki et al., 1997; Taylor et al., 1949). The mechanism(s) of elevated exercise heart rate after BR may represent one or a combination of several factors. It is possible that increased sympathetic nerve activity during maximal exercise contributes to BR-induced elevation in maximal heart rate since there is greater plasma norepinephrine concentrations during maximal exercise after BR (Engelke and Convertino, 1996). In addition, the heart rate response to a 0.02 μg/kg/min steady-state dose of isoproterenol is increased significantly after BR (Convertino et al., 1997), suggesting that cardiac β-adrenergic receptor sensitivity may be increased by confinement to bed. Therefore, increased sympathetic nerve activity and sensitivity of cardiac adrenergic receptors can explain, at least in part, elevated maximal heart rate after exposure to BR. However, despite increased heart rate, cardiac output during submaximal and maximal exercise is decreased following BR (Convertino, 1997; Hung et al., 1983; Saltin et al., 1968).

Mechanisms for maximal stroke volume. Because maximal heart rate is elevated following BR, it is clear that the reduction in maximal cardiac output and $\dot{V}O_{2\,max}$ is the result of a dramatic reduction in stroke volume. In a landmark investigation on the effects of BR, Saltin and co-workers (1968) demonstrated a 26% reduction in $\dot{V}O_{2\,max}$ in five young male subjects after they had been confined for 21 days in bed. The magnitude of the decrease of anaerobic power in this group of subjects was similar to a 26% reduction in maximal cardiac output from 20.0 l/min before to 14.8 l/min after BR. A compensatory elevation in maximal heart rate from 193 bpm before to 197 bpm after BR failed to compensate for an average reduction

Table 2.1 Mean changes in maximal oxygen uptake during bed rest without remedial procedures

References	BR, days	N	Subjects		$\dot{V}O_{2\,max}$, l/min		
			Age	Gender	Pre	Post	%Δ
Friman (1979)	7	22	25±1	M	3.30	3.11	−5.8
White et al. (1966)	10	3	21−26	M	3.66	3.47	−5.2
Convertino et al. (1982b)	10	12	45−55	M	2.03	1.91	−5.9
Convertino et al. (1982b)	10	12	45−55	M	2.15	1.81	−15.8
Convertino et al. (1986a)	10	15	45−65	M	2.74	2.52	−8.0
Convertino et al. (1986a)	10	17	45−65	F	1.61	1.49	−7.5
Convertino et al. (1986b)	10	10	36−51	M	2.42	2.25	−7.0
Convertino et al. (1987)	10	10	36−48	M	2.52	2.30	−8.7
Convertino (1998)	10	10	35−51	M	2.87	2.41	−16.0
Convertino (1998)	10	10	35−51	M	2.40	2.24	−6.7
Georgievskiy et al. (1966)	13	4	22−25	M	3.14	2.87	−8.6
Lamb et al. (1964)	14	8	24−34	M	2.43	2.26	−7.0
Convertino et al. (1977)	14	15	19−23	M	3.52	3.20	−9.1
Stremel et al. (1976)	14	7	19−22	M	3.83	3.36	−12.3
Convertino et al. (1982c)	15	4	20−26	M	3.86	3.32	−14.0
Engelke and Convertino (1998)	16	7	28−49	M	2.70	2.30	−14.8
Convertino et al. (1977)	17	8	23−34	F	2.06	1.86	−9.7
Saltin et al. (1968)	20	5	19−21	M	3.30	2.43	−26.4
Kakurin et al. (1966)	20	4	22−24	M	3.10	2.70	−12.9
Kashihara et al. (1994)	20	6	20−23	M	2.82	2.42	−14.2
Kashihara et al. (1994)	20	5	19−21	F	2.55	2.22	−12.9
Suzuki et al. (1997)	20	10	19−25	M	2.89	2.53	−12.5
Suzuki et al. (1997)	20	5	19−24	F	2.19	1.85	−15.5
Stevens et al. (1966)	26	22	18−23	M	2.58	2.04	−20.9
Taylor et al. (1949)	28	2		M	3.85	3.16	−17.9
Meehan et al. (1966)	28	14	19−24	M	3.75	3.04	−18.9
Greenleaf et al. (1989)	28	5	32−42	M	3.27	2.60	−20.5
Lamb et al. (1964)	30	8	17−24	M	2.66	2.28	−14.3
Katkovskiy et al. (1974)	30	3	24−29	M	3.09	2.02	−34.6
Mean					2.87	2.48	−13.6

Note: BR, bed rest
Source: Modified from Convertino (1995).

in stroke volume from 104 to 74 ml. The absence of a change in arteriovenous oxygen difference suggested that a primary mechanism for reduction in aerobic power associated with the deconditioning effects of BR was a severely compromised stroke volume.

Echocardiographic measurements demonstrated lower resting heart volume in subjects after BR (Kashihara et al., 1994; Levine et al., 1997; Saltin et al., 1968). It was subsequently proposed that reduced stroke volume and lower cardiac volume in subjects performing supine as well as upright exercise during BR may reflect decreased ventricular performance resulting from myocardial atrophy or other deterioration (Saltin et al., 1968). Recent evidence indicated that at least a portion of the reduction in heart volume after BR was associated with cardiac atrophy (Levine et al., 1997). To test the hypothesis that cardiac atrophy and its functional deterioration might contribute to reduced stroke volume during exercise, cardiac output and stroke volume were measured during submaximal and maximal exercise with radionuclide imaging in 12 middle-aged men before and after 10 days of BR (Hung et al., 1983). In confirmation of previous results (Saltin et al., 1968), a 17% reduction in $\dot{V}O_{2\,max}$ resulted from a 23% reduction in cardiac output (19.7 l/min before to 15.1 l/min after BR) with little change in the arteriovenous O_2 difference. The reduction in cardiac output was due solely to a 28% decrease in stroke volume since maximal heart rate increased from 170 bpm before to 180 bpm after BR. Despite a significant reduction in exercise stroke volume after BR, the ejection fraction actually increased at rest and during exercise (Hung et al., 1983). This increased ejection fraction after BR suggests that ventricular performance was maintained and that functional myocardial deterioration was not evident.

A reduced cardiac output in the presence of increased ejection fraction and heart rate during exercise after BR suggests that changes in venous return and cardiac filling probably represented a primary mechanism by which maximal stroke volume is reduced. Indeed, lower stroke volume and cardiac output have been associated with lower blood volume and cardiac filling (central venous) pressure during BR (Convertino et al., 1994; Saltin et al., 1968). Since venous return and cardiac filling limit maximal stroke volume (Frank–Starling relationship), the cardiac response to maximal exercise after BR shifts to a lower stroke volume. However, stroke volume remains higher at any given filling pressure after confinement to BR for less than two weeks (Convertino, 1997) suggesting that increased cardiac compliance may represent a mechanism to defend stroke volume in the presence of hypovolemia and reduced cardiac filling pressure. Unfortunately, there is evidence that exposure to BR for durations longer than two weeks without physical activity results in reduced myocardial compliance, which limits cardiac filling (Levine et al., 1997).

Since limited cardiac filling cannot be explained by myocardial mechanics during the initial two or more weeks of BR, a primary mechanism associated with reduced stroke volume during maximal exercise is lower circulating blood (plasma) volume. This hypothesis is supported by the close relationship between the magnitude of change in blood volume and $\dot{V}O_{2\,max}$ (Convertino, 1997). The time course of reduction in $\dot{V}O_{2\,max}$ shows a steep decline within the first few days of BR followed by a more gradual reduction thereafter (Georgiyevski et al., 1966; Greenleaf et al., 1989), which is similar to the time course of hypovolemia (Convertino et al., 1990; Greenleaf et al., 1989). Cross-sectional comparison of the data from 12 independent investigations demonstrated a high correlation between percent change in plasma volume and $\dot{V}O_{2\,max}$ (Convertino, 1997). The square of this correlation coefficient suggests that approximately 70% of the variability in $\dot{V}O_{2\,max}$ can be explained by lower plasma volume. Relative changes in plasma volume and $\dot{V}O_{2\,max}$ following 10 days of BR were assessed in 10 sedentary ($\dot{V}O_{2\,max} = 38$ ml$\cdot$kg$^{-1}\cdot$min^{-1}) and 10 moderately fit subjects ($\dot{V}O_{2\,max} = 49\ ml \cdot kg^{-1} \cdot min^{-1}$) in a longitudinal study (Convertino, 1998). A 16% reduction in $\dot{V}O_{2\,max}$ observed in the fit subjects was nearly three times that of the 6% decrease in the unfit group. These relative losses in aerobic capacity were matched by 16% and 6% reductions in blood volume in the fit and unfit groups, respectively. These findings reinforce the notion that the larger cardiovascular reserve associated with greater levels of physical fitness is usually associated with greater absolute reduction in that reserve after BR deconditioning (Convertino, 1986, 1997; Convertino et al., 1986a, 1998; Saltin et al., 1968). The correlation coefficient of 0.79 between the percent changes in plasma volume and $\dot{V}O_{2\,max}$ using individual data of all of our 20 subjects was similar to that of 0.84 generated from the 12 independent investigations (Convertino, 1997), suggesting that reduction in plasma volume contributes significantly to the limitation of maximal stroke volume, cardiac output, and $\dot{V}O_2$ during BR. This proposed cause–effect relationship is supported by the observation that plasma volume retention by daily exposure to orthostatic pressure gradients or intense exercise training during BR minimizes or eliminates the reduction in $\dot{V}O_{2\,max}$ (Convertino et al., 1982c; Greenleaf et al., 1989).

In addition to the effects of hypovolemia, reduced cardiac filling and stroke volume during exercise following BR could be accentuated by increased venous pooling in the lower extremities, since venous compliance of the legs increases by 20 to 25% during BR (Convertino et al., 1989); several observations support this. Despite maximal muscle pumping action on peripheral veins, increased leg venous pooling from application of lower body negative pressure caused lower central venous pressure, stroke volume, and cardiac output during exercise (Mack et al., 1988). Furthermore, reduction in $\dot{V}O_{2\,max}$ (~17%) after 10 days of BR in the upright posture was more than twice that in the supine posture (~7%) in spite of the same elevation in heart rate (Convertino et al., 1982b; 1983); and $\dot{V}O_2$ kinetics were significantly slowed in the upright compared to the supine posture (Convertino et al., 1984). That increased venous compliance may contribute to the reduction in post-BR cardiac filling, stroke volume and $\dot{V}O_{2\,max}$ is further supported by the observation that reduction in maximal stroke volume after BR was greater in the upright posture (Hung et al., 1983), whereas heart rate elevation in the upright posture was similar to that in the supine posture (Convertino et al., 1982a).

Peripheral mechanisms of oxygen delivery and utilization. The reduction in supine $\dot{V}O_{2\,max}$ supports the hypothesis that peripheral mechanisms controlling $A-\dot{V}O_2$ difference, i.e., regional oxygen delivery and utilization, probably contribute to reduction in aerobic power following BR. Maximal oxygen utilization by exercising muscle may be compromised by reduction in oxidative enzyme function (Hikida et al., 1989) and greater accumulation of blood lactate (Convertino et al., 1986b; Saltin et al., 1968; Williams and Convertino, 1988) in addition to the reduced capacity to deliver oxygen to skeletal muscle. In addition to the direct effect of reduced blood volume on cardiac filling and output, prolonged BR deconditioning can decrease red blood cell mass by 5% to 25% beyond 2–3 weeks of BR (Convertino et al., 1981, 1982b, 1984; Lamb et al., 1964; White et al., 1966), which may contribute to reduced $\dot{V}O_{2\,max}$ by compromising blood oxygen-carrying capacity. However, the correlation between changes in red cell mass and the $\dot{V}O_{2\,max}$ is low and the reduction in $\dot{V}O_{2\,max}$ with BR can occur without change in red cell mass (Convertino et al., 1986b). In general, hematocrit remains constant or increases during BR, suggesting that oxygen-carrying capacity per unit of blood should not change. Therefore, it is unclear if decreased red cell mass induced by BR is a factor for reduction in the maximal capacity to deliver oxygen to active muscle.

Peripheral mechanisms for muscle blood flow. In addition to the reduction in red cell mass, confinement to bed is associated with lower resting blood flow in leg muscles (Convertino et al., 1989a) and a reduction in capillarization in the muscular bed (Hikida et al., 1989). These changes are consistent with reductions in maximal conductance and fatiguability in calf muscles after 16 days of BR that were correlated significantly to the magnitude of the decrease in $\dot{V}O_{2\,max}$ (Engelke and Convertino, 1998). Although changes in peripheral mechanisms associated with restricted delivery to and utilization of oxygen by skeletal muscle could contribute to lower $\dot{V}O_{2\,max}$ after BR, this mechanism has not been apparent when based on calculation of maximal A$-\dot{V}O_2$ difference (Hung et al., 1983; Saltin et al., 1968). It is probable that the limitation of cardiac output is such an overwhelming limiting factor that peripheral mechanisms are relatively insignificant. However, if blood volume and cardiac filling are not fully limiting, it is probable that the influence of peripheral mechanisms for limiting $\dot{V}O_{2\,max}$ may become more apparent.

DECONDITIONING RESULTS FROM SPACEFLIGHT

As a result of operational and logistical limitations in the spaceflight environment, there are few data on the $\dot{V}O_{2\,max}$ of astronauts. $\dot{V}O_{2\,max}$ was measured before spaceflight and immediately after return to Earth in six astronauts (four men and two women, age 35–50 yr) who participated on two US Spacelab Life Sciences missions (Levine et al., 1996). The duration of the spaceflight was either 9 (N = 3) or 14 days (N = 3). Average $\dot{V}O_{2\,max}$ of these six astronauts was reduced by 22% immediately after flight. Similar to BR, spaceflight is associated with reduced plasma and blood volume (Convertino, 1995, 1996; Fischer et al., 1967; Johnson et al., 1977), higher heart rates, and lower cardiac filling and output (Atkov et al., 1987; Convertino, 1990; Levine et al., 1996; Yegorov et al., 1981). In the absence of evidence for deterioration in myocardial function (Atkov et al., 1987; Henry et al., 1977; Yegorov et al., 1981), the reduced stroke volume, cardiac output, and $\dot{V}O_{2\,max}$ associated with spaceflight can most likely be attributed to reduced circulating blood volume and its effect on central venous filling pressure and venous return, to ventricular filling, and to cardiovascular hemodynamics rather than impairment of cardiac function. In addition, reduction in oxidative enzyme activity in skeletal muscle (Edgerton et al., 1995) could contribute to lower $\dot{V}O_{2\,max}$ by limiting oxygen extraction and utilization by working muscle.

The potential operational consequence of reduced aerobic reserve is the inability to maintain physical work requirements during spaceflight for a given period of time, i.e., lower endurance. This was supported by decreased endurance to a standardized exercise test (125 watts for 5 min) in the two crew members during the early part of a 96-day flight aboard the Russian Salyut-6 space station; it was manifested by increased heart rate, elevated arterial pressure, reduced stroke volume, and an inability to complete the 5-min exercise bout on the 24th day of flight (Georgiyevskiy et al., 1980). Clearly, the lower gravitational stress in space crews produced by the space environment mainifested itself as greater physiological deconditioning during the course of the space mission.

RECONDITIONING EFFECTS

Data from the BR study of Saltin and co-workers (1968) are often cited as evidence favoring the use of exercise programs as an effective technique for enhancing the recovery from the deconditioning effects on $\dot{V}O_{2\,max}$ following BR. In three of their habitually sedentary subjects, $\dot{V}O_{2\,max}$ levels were restored within 10 to 14 days of recovery from BR. However, their two habitually active subjects required 30 to 40 days of physical activity to restore their $\dot{V}O_{2\,max}$ values to pre-BR levels. These data suggest that exercise training following BR deconditioning is instrumental for enhancing the recovery rate of $\dot{V}O_{2\,max}$. However, a limitation of this suggestion is that the study was not designed to distinguish between the effects of exercise reconditioning, and those of resumption of usual activities in the normal upright posture; all five subjects underwent exercise training. In a study designed to address this issue (DeBusk et al., 1983), $\dot{V}O_{2\,max}$ was compared in six subjects who performed prescribed physical exercise daily for 60 days after 10 days of BR (exercise group) and six subjects who simply resumed their customary ambulatory activities (control group). Despite significantly greater increase in the exercise group's $\dot{V}O_{2\,max}$ at 60 days when compared to the control group, $\dot{V}O_{2\,max}$ of both groups returned to pre-BR levels by 30 days after BR. These data indicate that simple resumption of normal physical activities after BR was as effective as formal exercise conditioning for restoring their functional capacity to baseline levels. Further supporting data demonstrate that a randomized trial of in-hospital exercise conditioning did not increase treadmill performance (Sivarajan et al., 1981); and that $\dot{V}O_{2\,max}$ was restored by 14 days of recovery from a 10-day BR (Convertino et al., 1985), and by 30 days of recovery from 7 days of BR (Friman, 1979) in subjects who merely resumed ambulatory activities with no additional daily exercise training. Thus, resumption of normal, ambulatory activity appears adequate for reconditioning and formal exercise training of high intensity may accelerate this process, especially following longer deconditioning periods.

The most effective countermeasure for overcoming deconditioning $\dot{V}O_{2\,max}$ is exercise training during BR or spaceflight. The data in Table 2.2 ($\Delta\dot{V}O_{2\,max}$ with remedial procedures) indicate that the average reduction in $\dot{V}O_{2\,max}$ during BR can be ameliorated by exercise training to one-third of that expected by BR alone (Table 2.1, $\Delta\dot{V}O_{2\,max}$ without remedial procedures). Results from the US Skylab IV mission corroborate the prevention of deconditioning effects on aerobic capacity with exercise training by demonstrating that the $\dot{V}O_{2\,max}$ of all 3 astronauts actually increased by 8% after 79 to 83 days of flight (Convertino, 1990, 1995). However, the

Table 2.2   Effect of exercise training during bed rest on maximal oxygen uptake

References	BR, days	N	Age	Gender	Pre	Post	%Δ	Min/day	Training schedule intensity	Training mode
			Subjects		$\dot{V}O_{2max}$, l/min					
Convertino (1987)	10	10	36–48	M	3.25	3.21	−1.2	~15 (last day)	100% $\dot{V}O_{2max}$	CE SUP
Stremel et al. (1976)	14	7	19–22	M	3.80	3.45	−9.2	60	68% $\dot{V}O_{2max}$	CE SUP
Stremel et al. (1976)	14	7	19–22	M	3.77	3.59	−4.8	60	21% peak torque	RES SUP
Chase et al. (1966)	15	4	22–26	M	3.19	3.42	7.2	30	71% $\dot{V}O_{2max}$	CE SUP
Chase et al. (1966)	15	4	21–24	M	2.96	3.42	15.5	30	76% $\dot{V}O_{2max}$	TRAMP SUP
Kashihara et al. (1994)	20	3	20	M	3.20	2.84	−11.3	60	40% $\dot{V}O_{2max}$	CE UP
Rodahl et al. (1967)	24	2	19–20	M	3.00	2.80	−6.7	60	50% $\dot{V}O_{2max}$	CE SUP
Rodahl et al. (1967)	24	2	18–19	M	2.80	2.80	0.0	60	50% $\dot{V}O_{2max}$	CE UP
Miller et al. (1965)	28	6	18–21	M	2.91	2.28	−21.6	60	30% $\dot{V}O_{2max}$	CE SUP
Chase et al. (1966)	30	4	21–25	M	3.17	2.92	−7.9	45	75% $\dot{V}O_{2max}$	TRAMP SUP
Chase et al. (1966)	30	4	21–22	M	3.51	3.19	−9.1	15	75% $\dot{V}O_{2max}$	TRAMP SUP
Greenleaf et al. (1989)	30	7	32–42	M	3.13	3.14	0.3	60	90% $\dot{V}O_{2max}$	CE SUP
Greenleaf et al. (1989)	30	7	32–42	M	3.24	2.90	−10.5	60	100% peak torque	ISOK SUP
Mean					3.23	3.07	−4.6			

Note: BR, bed rest; CE, cycle ergometer; TM, treadmill; UP, upright position; SUP, supine position.
Source: Modified from Convertino (1995).

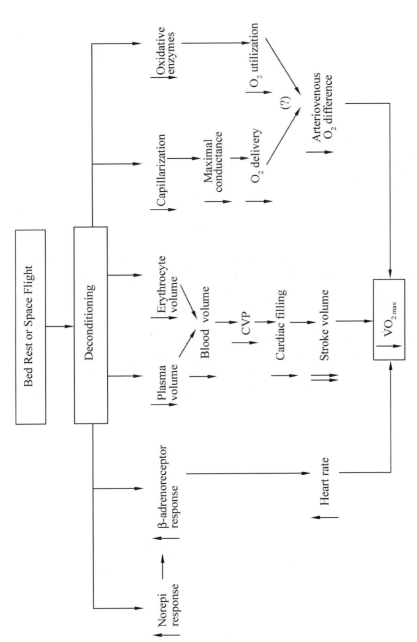

Figure 2.1 Cardiovascular mechanisms contributing to changes in maximal oxygen uptake ($\dot{V}O_{2\,max}$) during bed rest or spaceflight.

exercise quality appears important for assessing effects of prescribed physical activity for minimizing reduction in $\dot{V}O_{2\,max}$ during BR. For instance, dynamic aerobic exercise training was ineffective when exercise intensity was less than 40% $\dot{V}O_{2\,max}$ (Kashihara et al., 1994; Miller et al., 1965). Isokinetic resistive exercise training was also less effective for ameliorating the reduction in $\dot{V}O_{2\,max}$ after BR (Greenleaf et al., 1989). Thus, exercise training performed during BR can ameliorate the reduction in $\dot{V}O_{2\,max}$ when exercise intensity is greater than 40% $\dot{V}O_{2\,max}$ and the training protocol is designed to challenge aerobic metabolic demands.

OVERVIEW

Deconditioning effects of BR or spaceflight on the cardiovascular system can be divided into central (cardiac) and peripheral mechanisms that contribute to maintenance of $\dot{V}O_{2\,max}$ (Figure 2.1). An increased maximal heart rate is associated with elevations in sympathetic activity (norepinephrine release) at maximal exercise and increased cardiac β-adrenergic response. These adrenergic responses could also increase cardiac contractility, which would increase ejection fraction during exercise following deconditioning even with reductions in stroke volume and cardiac filling. Despite elevated maximal heart rate and probable cardiac contractility, maximal cardiac output is reduced dramatically by a significant decrease in stroke volume. Since cardiac contractility is probably enhanced, the lowered stroke volume must be due primarily to reduced cardiac filling associated with lower blood volume. Increased compliance of veins in leg muscles may also contribute to the limited venous return, especially after return to the upright posture. Although arteriovenous O_2 difference has been reported unaltered following BR and spaceflight, reductions in oxidative enzymes, capillarization, and maximal blood flow in the muscle could limit oxygen delivery and utilization. The ultimate consequence of these alterations in cardiac and vascular functions resulting from BR or spaceflight deconditioning is reduction in aerobic power.

REFERENCES

Atkov, O. Y., Bednenko, V. S., and Fomina, G. A. (1987) Ultrasound techniques in space medicine. *Aviat. Space Environ. Med.* **58**(Suppl. 9): A69–A73.

Chase, G. A., Grave, C., and Rowell, L. B. (1966) Independence of changes in functional and performance capacities attending prolonged bed rest. *Aerospace Med.* **37**: 1232–1238.

Convertino, V. A. (1983) Effect of orthostatic stress on exercise performance after bed rest: relation to inhospital rehabilitation. *J. Cardiac Rehabil.* **3**: 660–663.

Convertino, V. A. (1986) Exercise responses after inactivity. In: *Inactivity: Physiological Effects*, edited by H. Sandler and J. Vernikos-Danellis. Orlando, FL: Academic Press, pp. 149–191.

Convertino, V. A. (1987) Potential benefits of maximal exercise just prior to return from weightlessness. *Aviat. Space Environ. Med.* **58**: 568–572.

Convertino, V. A. (1990) Physiological adaptations to weightlessness: effects on exercise and work performance. *Exerc. Sport Sci. Rev.* **18**: 119–165.

Convertino, V. A. (1995) Exercise and adaptation to microgravity environments. In: Fregly, M. J., and Blatteis, C. M., eds. *Handbook of Physiology: Environmental Physiology. III. The Gravitational Environment.* New York: Oxford University Press. Section 1, Chap. 36, pp. 815–843.

Convertino, V. A. (1996) Clinical aspects of the control of plasma volume at microgravity and during return to one gravity. *Med. Sci. Sports Exerc.* **28**: S45–S52.

Convertino, V. A. (1997) Cardiovascular consequences of bed rest: effects on maximal oxygen uptake. *Med. Sci. Sports Exerc.* **29**: 191–196.

Convertino, V. A. (1998) Changes in maximal oxygen uptake and plasma volume in fit and unfit subjects following exposure to a simulation of microgravity. *Acta Physiol. Scand.* **164**: 251–257.

Convertino, V. A., Bisson, R., Bates, R., Goldwater, D., and Sandler, H. (1981) Effects of anti-orthostatic bed rest on the cardiorespiratory responses to exercise. *Aviat. Space Environ. Med.* **52**: 251–255.

Convertino, V. A., Doerr, D. F., Eckberg, D. L., Fritsch, J. M., and Vernikos-Danellis, J. (1990) Head-down bed rest impairs vagal baroreflex responses and provokes orthostatic hypotension. *J. Appl. Physiol.* **68**: 1458–1464.

Convertino, V. A., Doerr, D. F., Ludwig, D. A., and Vernikos, J. (1994) Effect of simulated microgravity on cardiopulmonary baroreflex control of forearm vascular resistance. *Am. J. Physiol. Regulatory Integrative Comp. Physiol.* **266**: R1962–R1969.

Convertino, V. A., Doerr, D. F., Mathes, K. L., Stein, S. L., and Buchanan, P. (1989) Changes in volume, muscle compartment, and compliance of the lower extremities in man following 30 days of exposure to simulated microgravity. *Aviat. Space Environ. Med.* **60**: 653–658.

Convertino, V. A., Doerr, D. F., and Stein, S. L. (1989) Changes in size and compliance of the calf following 30 days of simulated microgravity. *J. Appl. Physiol.* **66**: 1509–1512.

Convertino, V. A., Goldwater, D. J., and Sandler, H. (1982a) Effect of orthostatic stress on exercise performance after bed rest. *Aviat. Space Environ. Med.* **53**: 652–657.

Convertino, V. A., Goldwater, D. J., and Sandler, H. (1984) $\dot{V}O_2$ kinetics of constant-load exercise following bed rest-induced deconditioning. *J. Appl. Physiol.* **57**: 1545–1550.

Convertino, V. A., Goldwater, D. J., and Sandler, H. (1986a) Bed rest-induced peak $\dot{V}O_2$ reduction associated with age, gender and aerobic capacity. *Aviat. Space Environ. Med.* **57**: 17–22.

Convertino, V. A., Hung, J., Goldwater, D. J., and DeBusk, R. F. (1982b) Cardiovascular responses to exercise in middle-aged men following ten days of bed rest. *Circulation* **65**: 134–140.

Convertino, V. A., Karst, G. M., Kirby, C. R., and Goldwater, D. J. (1986b) Effect of simulated weightlessness on exercise-induced anaerobic threshold. *Aviat. Space Environ. Med.* **57**: 325–331.

Convertino, V. A., Kirby, C. R., Karst, G. M., and Goldwater, D. J. (1985) Responses to muscular exercise following repeated simulated weightlessness. *Aviat. Space Environ. Med.* **56**: 540–546.

Convertino, V. A., Polet, J. L., Engelke, K. A., Hoffler, G. W., Lane, L. D., and Blomqvist, C. G. (1997) Evidence for increased β-adrenoreceptor responsiveness induced by 14 days of simulated microgravity in humans. *Am. J. Physiol. Regulatory Integrative Comp. Physiol.* **273**: R93–R99.

Convertino, V. A., Sandler, H., Webb, P., and Annis, J. F. (1982c) Induced venous pooling and cardiorespiratory responses to exercise after bed rest. *J. Appl. Physiol.* **52**: 1343–1348.

Convertino, V. A., Stremel, R. W., Bernauer, E. M., and Greenleaf, J. E. (1977) Cardiorespiratory responses to exercise after bed rest in men and women. *Acta Astronautica* **4**: 895–905.

DeBusk, R. F., Convertino, V. A., Hung, J., and Goldwater, D. (1983) Exercise conditioning in middle-aged men after 10 days of bed rest. *Circulation* **68**: 245–250.

Deitrick, J. E., Whedon, G. D., Shorr, E., Toscani, V., and Davis, V. B. (1948) Effects of immobilization upon various metabolic and physiologic functions of normal men. *Am. J. Med.* **4**: 3–35.

Edgerton, V. R., Zhou, M.-Y., Ohira, Y., Klitgaard, H., Jiang, B., Bell, G., Harris, B., Saltin, B., Gollnick, P. D., Roy, R. R., Day, M. K., and Greenisen, M. (1995) Human fiber size and enzymatic properties after 5 and 11 days of spaceflight. *J. Appl. Physiol.* **78**: 1733–1739.

Engelke, K. A., and Convertino, V. A. (1996) Catecholamine response to maximal exercise following 16 days of simulated microgravity. *Aviat. Space Environ. Med.* **67**: 243–247.

Engelke, K. A., and Convertino, V. A. (1998) Restoration of peak vascular conductance after simulated microgravity by maximal exercise. *Clin. Physiol.* **18**: 544–553.

Fischer, C. L., Johnson, P. C., and Berry, C. A. (1967) Red blood cell and plasma volume changes in manned spaceflight. *J. A. M. A.* **200**: 579–583.

Friman, G. (1979) Effect of clinical bed rest for seven days on physical performance. *Acta Med. Scand.* **205**: 389–393.

Georgiyevskiy, V. S., Kakurin, L. I., Katkovskii, B. S., and Senkevich, Y. A. (1966) Maximum oxygen consumption and functional state of the circulation in simulated zero gravity. In: *The Oxygen Regime of the Organism and its Regulation*, edited by N. V. Lauer and A. Z. Kilchinskaya, Kiev: Naukova Dumka, pp. 181–184.

Georgiyevskiy, V. S., Lapshina, N. A., Andriyako, L. Y., Umnova, L. V., Doroshev, V. G., Alferova, I. V., Ragozin, V. N., and Kobzev, Y. A. (1980) Circulation in exercising crew members of the first main expedition aboard Salyut-6. *Kosm. Biol. Aviakosm. Med.* **14**(3): 15–18.

Greenleaf, J. E., Bernauer, E. M., Ertl, A. C., Trowbridge, T. S., and Wade, C. E. (1989) Work capacity during 30 days of bed rest with isotonic and isokinetic exercise training. *J. Appl. Physiol.* **67**: 1820–1826.

Greenleaf, J. E., and Kozlowski, S. (1982a) Physiological consequences of reduced physical activity during bed rest. *Exerc. Sport Sci. Rev.* **10**: 83–119.

Greenleaf, J. E., and Kozlowski, S. (1982b) Reduction in peak oxygen uptake after prolonged bed rest. *Med. Sci. Sports Exerc.* **14**: 477–480.

Henry, W. L., Epstein, S. E., Griffith, J. M., Goldstein, R. E., and Redwood, D. R. (1977) Effect of prolonged space flight on cardiac function and dimensions. In: Johnston, R. S., and Dietlein, L. F., eds. *Biomedical Results from Skylab*, Washington, DC: National Aeronautics and Space Administration, pp. 366–371.

Hikida, R. S., Gollnick, P. D., Dudley, G. A., Convertino, V. A., and Buchanan, P. (1989) Structural and metabolic characteristics of human skeletal muscle following 30 days of simulated microgravity. *Aviat. Space Environ. Med.* **60**: 664–670.

Hung, J., Goldwater, D., Convertino, V. A., McKillop, J. H., Goris, M. L., and DeBusk, R. F. (1983) Mechanisms for decreased exercise capacity following bed rest in normal middle-aged men. *Am. J. Cardiol.* **51**: 344–348.

Johnson, P. C., Driscoll, T. B., and LeBlanc, A. D. (1977) Blood volume changes. In: Johnston, R. S. and Dietlein, L. F., eds. *Biomedical Results from Skylab*, Washington, DC: National Aeronautics and Space Administration, pp. 235–241.

Kakurin, L. I., Akhrem-Adhremovich, R. M., Vanyushina, Y. V., Varbaronov, R. A., Georgiyevskii, V. S., Kotkovskiy, B. S., Kotovskaya, A. R., Mukharlyamov, N. M., Panferova, N. Y., Pushkar, Y. T., Senkevich, Y. A., Simpura, S. F., Cherpakhin, M. A., and Shamrov, P. G. (1966) The influence of restricted muscular activity on man's endurance of physical stress, accelerations and orthostatics. In: *Soviet Conference on Space Biology and Medicine*, Moscow, pp. 110–117.

Kashihara, H., Haruna, Y., Suzuki, Y., Kawakuba, K., Takenaka, K., Bonde-Petersen, F., and Gunji, A. (1994) Effects of mild supine exercise during 20 days bed rest on maximal oxygen uptake rate in young humans. *Acta Physiol. Scand.* **150** (Suppl. 616): 19–26.

Katkovskiy, B. S., Machinskiy, G. V., Toman, P. S., Danilova, V. I., and Demida, B. F. (1974) Man's physical performance after thirty-day hypokinesia with countermeasures. *Kosm. Biol. Med.* **8**(4): 43–47.

Lamb, L. E., Johnson, R. L., Stevens, P. M., and Welch, B. E. (1964) Cardiovascular deconditioning from space cabin simulator confinement. *Aerospace Med.* **35**: 420–428.

Levine, B. D., Lane, L. D., Watenpaugh, D. E., Gaffney, F. A., Buckey, J. C., and Blomqvist, C. G. (1996) Maximal exercise performance after adaptation to microgravity. *J. Appl. Physiol.* **81**: 686–694.

Levine, B. D., Zuckerman, J. H., and Pawilczyk, J. A. (1997) Cardiac atrophy after bed-rest deconditioning: a nonneural mechanism for orthostatic intolerance. *Circulation* **96**: 517–525.

Mack, G., Nose, H., and Nadel, E. R. (1988) Role of cardiopulmonary baroreflexes during dynamic exercise. *J. Appl. Physiol.* **65**: 1827–1832.

Meehan, J. P., Henry, J. P., Brunjes, S., and DeVries, H. (1966) *Investigation to determine the effects of long-term bed rest on G-tolerance and on psychomotor performance.* Los Angeles, CA: Dep. of Physiology, University of Southern California, (NASA-CR-62073).

Miller, P. B., Johnson, R. L., and Lamb, L. E. (1965) Effects of moderate physical exercise during four weeks of bed rest on circulatory functions in man. *Aerospace Med.* **36**: 1077–1082.

Rodahl, K., Birkhead, N. C., Blizzard, J. J., Issekutz, B., Jr., and Pruett, E. D. R. (1967) Physiological changes during prolonged bed rest. In: *Nutrition and Physical Activity,* edited by G. Blix. Uppsala: Almqvist & Wiksells, pp. 107–113.

Saltin, B., Blomqvist, G., Mitchell, J. H., Johnson, R. L., Wildenthal, K., and Chapman, C. B. (1968) Response to exercise after bed rest and after training. *Circulation* **38**(Suppl 7): 1–78.

Sivarajan, E. S., Bruce, R. A., Almes, M. J., Green, B., Belanger, L., Lindskog, B. D., Newton, K. M., and Mansfield, L. W. (1981) In-hospital exercise after myocardial infarction does not improve treadmill performance. *N. Engl. J. Med.* **305**: 357–362.

Stevens, P. M., Miller, P. B., Gilbert, C. A., Lynch, T. N., Johnson, R. L., and Lamb, L. E. (1966) Influence of long-term lower body negative pressure on the circulatory function of man during prolonged bed rest. *Aerospace Med.* **37**: 357–367.

Stremel, R. W., Convertino, V. A., Bernauer, E. M., and Greenleaf, J. E. (1976) Cardiorespiratory deconditioning with static and dynamic leg exercise during bed rest. *J. Appl. Physiol.* **41**: 905–909.

Suzuki, Y., Iwamoto, S., Haruna, Y., Kuriyama, K., Kawakubo, K., and Gunji, A. (1997) Effects of 20 days horizontal bed rest on mechanical efficiency during steady state exercise at mild-moderate intensities in young subjects. *J. Gravitat. Physiol.* **4**: S46–S52.

Taylor, H. L., Henschel, A., Brozek, J., and Keys, A. (1949) Effects of bed rest on cardiovascular function and work performance. *J. Appl. Physiol.* **2**: 223–239.

White, P. D., Nyberg, J. W., and White, W. J. (1966) A comparative study of the physiological effects of immersion and recombency. In: *Proceedings of the 2nd Annual Biomedical Research Conference,* Houston, TX, pp. 117–166.

Williams, D. A., and Convertino, V. A. (1988) Circulating lactate and FFA during exercise: Effect of reduction in plasma volume following simulated microgravity. *Aviat. Space Environ. Med.* **59**: 1042–1046.

Yegorov, A. D., Itsekhovskiy, O. G., Polyakova, A. P., Turchaninova, V. F., Alferova, I. V., Savelyeva, V. G., Domracheva, M. V., Batenchuk-Tusko, T. V., Doroshev, V. G., and Kobzev, Y. A. (1981) Results of studies of hemodynamics and phase structure of the cardiac cycle during functional test with graded exercise during 140-day flight aboard the Salyut-6 station. *Kosm. Biol. Aviakosm. Med.* **15**(3): 18–22.

CHAPTER 3

Physiological Consequences of Deconditioning in Physically Active Populations

James E. Graves, Lori L. Ploutz-Snyder, and Michael L. Pollock[†]

Department of Health and Physical Education, Syracuse University, Syracuse, New York, USA

> Exercise cannot secure us from that dissolution to which we are decreed; but while the soul and body continue united, it can make the association pleasing, and give probable hopes that they shall be disjoined by an easy separation... to die is the fate of man; but to die with lingering anguish is generally his folly.
>
> *Samuel Johnson*

INTRODUCTION

Physically active individuals enjoy a variety of health and fitness benefits that foster disease prevention, improve functional capacity of the body, and enhance the quality of life. Specific health benefits include reduced incidence of cardiovascular disease, colon cancer, obesity, diabetes, and osteoporosis, and improved mental health (U.S. Department of Health and Human Services, 1996). Specific fitness benefits include development and maintenance of cardiorespiratory capacity, muscular strength and endurance, flexibility, and a healthy level of body composition. These improvements in physical fitness enhance one's ability to complete the activities of daily living, preserve the maintenance of independent living, reduce risk of falling in the elderly, and contribute to athletic performance at all levels of competition.

[†]Deceased

Physiological adaptations that result from participation in physical activity are specific to the type of activity performed (McArdle et al., 1991). Aerobic exercise training (e.g., walking, jogging, stair-climbing) develops cardiorespiratory capacity and the ability to participate in continuous activity such as aerobic endurance exercise. Resistance exercises (weightlifting or calisthenics) are anaerobic and promote increased muscular strength (the ability to exert force), muscular endurance (resistance to fatigue), and the development and maintenance of muscle mass which contribute to a healthy body composition. In recognition of exercise specificity, exercise professionals recommend participation in a well-rounded exercise program that includes aerobic exercise training, resistance exercise training, and exercises that improve flexibility (American College of Sports Medicine, 1998).

A key tenet for improving physiologic function through participation in physical activity is the principle of overload: the requirement that physical activity be performed at a level greater than "normal" to induce adaptation (McArdle et al., 1991). Overload is achieved by manipulation of exercise mode (type), frequency, intensity (level), duration, and overall volume of activity (American College of Sports Medicine, 1998). A moderate progression of overload is required to elicit continued adaptation during a physical training program. In habitually active persons and elite athletes, continued progression may eventually result in increased risk of injury or "overtraining." These individuals may benefit most by exercising at a near-constant level to maintain a desired amount of fitness as opposed to progressing in their program, because further physical improvement in these people is usually minimal (Pollock and Wilmore, 1990).

The benefits of physical training are reversible (McArdle et al., 1991; Neufer, 1989). Continued participation at an appropriate level is required to maintain health status as well as functional capacity. It is generally recognized that the health and fitness benefits of physical activity can be maintained with reduced training frequency or reduced training volume as long as intensity (level) of the activity is not compromised (American College of Sports Medicine, 1998). This is true for aerobic as well as anaerobic activity. Physiologic function becomes compromised after a relatively short period of time following reduction in exercise training intensity or cessation of training (detraining).

The loss of physiological function during reduction in training intensity or detraining is deconditioning. Deconditioning also occurs in sedentary individuals during long-duration water immersion, spaceflight, and bed rest (Greenleaf, 1997). In recently trained individuals, deconditioning may lead to complete reversal of physiologic function to or even below pre-training, sedentary levels. In highly trained athletes some of the physiologic benefit of activity can be retained during deconditioning, although long-term (greater than 6 months) studies of deconditioning in highly trained populations have not been conducted.

In this chapter we will review the effects of deconditioning on physiological function in physically active populations. Studies of recently trained individuals will be considered as well as those that have employed long-term training, and those utilizing highly trained athletes. Most investigators have concentrated on loss of functional capacity and the responsible mechanisms during deconditioning. Few studies have addressed the influence of deconditioning on health status. The health and fitness benefits of participation in physical activity are related (American College of Sports Medicine, 1998), and protection from disease is probably decreased during deconditioning (Greenleaf et al., 1994). Following a description of the physiological consequences of detraining on aerobic and resistance exercise conditioning, we will discuss implications of prescription of exercise to physically active individuals in situations that might lead to deconditioning.

EFFECT OF DECONDITIONING ON AEROBIC EXERCISE TRAINING

Cardiovascular Consequences of Reduced Training

Aerobic exercise training results in increased ability to utilize oxygen to improve physical (aerobic) performance. Mechanisms associated with these changes include both cardiovascular and metabolic adaptations (Holloszy and Coyle, 1984). Cardio-vascular adaptations to aerobic exercise training indicate that the maximal volume of oxygen that can be consumed ($\dot{V}O_{2\,max}$ typically measured during incremental exercise to exhaustion) is increased by aerobic exercise training as a result of an increased ability of the heart to pump a greater volume of blood (cardiac output) and enhancement of exercising skeletal muscle to remove oxygen from the blood (Table 3.1). Maximal cardiac output increases primarily by an increase in stroke volume (Saltin, 1969). However, the unchanged cardiac output during a given level of submaximal exercise following training is achieved by a greater stroke volume and lower heart rate. In addition, the proportion of cardiac output delivered to exercising skeletal muscle following training increases because of increased vascularization of the capillary bed (Klausen et al., 1981). Increased intracellular myoglobin (Pattengale and Holloszy, 1967) and aerobic enzymes (Barnard et al., 1970; Kiessling, 1971) facilitate production of energy through aerobic metabolism.

Maximal oxygen uptake

Maximal oxygen uptake (aerobic capacity) can be maintained in previously trained individuals when training frequency (Hickson and Rosenkoetter, 1981) or duration (Hickson et al., 1982) are reduced by as much as two-thirds, as long as training intensity is maintained. When training intensity decreases by one-third, however, $\dot{V}O_{2\,max}$ declines dramatically (Hickson et al., 1985). Unfortunately, maintenance of aerobic capacity with training does not continue forever, even when training intensity is maintained. Pollock et al. (1997) studied 21 50-year-old elite track athletes for 20 years. Nine of those athletes who continued to train at high intensity showed a 15% reduction in $\dot{V}O_{2\,max}$ over the 20-year period. The reduction in aerobic capacity for those nine individuals, however, was significantly less than the 34% reduction observed in those who greatly reduced their training intensity.

Table 3.1   Cardiovascular adaptations to aerobic exercise training

Variables	Adaptation
Maximal values	
Oxygen uptake	↑
Cardiac output	↑
Heart rate	= or ↓
Stroke volume	↑
Arteriovenous oxygen difference	↑
Systolic blood pressure	=
Rate-pressure product	=
Endurance time	↑
Ejection fraction	↑
Submaximal values	
Oxygen uptake	= or ↓
Cardiac output	= or ↓
Heart rate	↓
Stroke volume	↑
Systolic blood pressure	↓
Rate-pressure product	↓
Resting values	
Oxygen uptake	=
Heart rate	↓
Systolic blood pressure	= or ↓
Diastolic blood pressure	= or ↓
Rate-pressure product	↓

Source: Adapted from Pollock and Wilmore (1990), p. 92.

The magnitude of decline in $\dot{V}O_{2\,max}$ during reduced training is related to the degree to which exercise intensity is compromised. A one-third reduction in training intensity resulted in a 4.2% to 5.8% decline in $\dot{V}O_{2\,max}$, whereas a two-thirds reduction in intensity resulted in a 9.5% to 25.8% decline (Hickson et al., 1985). Interestingly, most of the decrease in $\dot{V}O_{2\,max}$ occurs during the first 5 weeks of reduced training regardless of the magnitude of the change in intensity (Hickson et al., 1985).

In physically active individuals who stop training, $\dot{V}O_{2\,max}$ is reduced more rapidly. Coyle et al. (1984) reported a 7% reduction in $\dot{V}O_{2\,max}$ in highly trained distance runners and cyclists following just 12 days of detraining. This loss of aerobic capacity was accompanied by reduction in maximal cardiac output by 7%, in stroke volume by 10%, and in oxygen pulse by 11%. Aerobic capacity continued to decline by 16% following 84 days of detraining, a magnitude similar to that observed during bed rest deconditioning (Greenleaf, 1997). Thus, $\dot{V}O_{2\,max}$ following detraining in those previously highly trained individuals was still 17% greater than that found in sedentary controls after 84 days of detraining. The slope of the change in $\dot{V}O_{2\,max}$ from 56 days to 84 days of detraining was negative, however, indicating that detraining continuing beyond 84 days would likely result in a still further decline in aerobic capacity.

Complete return of $\dot{V}O_{2\,max}$ to pre-training values occurs after long-term (> 6 weeks) deconditioning in most populations including adult females (Fringer and Stull, 1974; Wang et al., 1997), adolescent males (Fournier et al., 1982), and adult males (Miyashita et al., 1978; Simoneau et al., 1987). Data from Ready and Quinney (1982) are an exception in that alterations in the "anaerobic threshold" in males after 9 weeks of endurance training (80% $\dot{V}O_{2\,max}$) resulted in incomplete return of aerobic capacity following 9 weeks of detraining. Moore et al. (1987) have also reported that when sedentary individuals participate in short-term (7 weeks), low-intensity training, the small gains in $\dot{V}O_{2\,max}$ may be retained for up to 3 weeks after training cessation.

The decline in $\dot{V}O_{2\,max}$ during detraining is a result of reduction in both cardiac output and arteriovenous O_2 difference (Coyle et al., 1984, 1985). Maximum cardiac output, however, is reduced within the first 12 days of detraining, whereas maximum arteriovenous O_2 difference can be maintained during at least 21 days of detraining (Coyle et al., 1985).

Heart rate

Since the heart rate (HR) of highly trained athletes at any relative (percent of maximal) exercise intensity (including the maximal level) increases during deconditioning (Coyle et al., 1984, 1985; Martin et al., 1986; Michael et al., 1972), the reduction in cardiac output must be caused by a decrease in stroke volume. In addition to a marked increase in maximal HR during deconditioning in highly trained athletes, HR recovery time increases following an acute bout of aerobic exercise (Michael et al., 1972). Previously trained individuals show little change in maximal HR during training (Pollock and Wilmore, 1990) or during subsequent deconditioning (Fournier et al., 1982; Fringer and Stull, 1974). Thus, the reduction in maximum cardiac output during deconditioning in previously trained individuals must also be caused by a decline in stroke volume.

Stroke volume

The reduction in stroke volume during deconditioning is associated with and may be caused in part by a decrease in heart mass. Ehsani et al. (1978) measured changes in left ventricular dimensions and mass after aerobic conditioning and deconditioning and observed complete loss of training-induced increases in ventricular volume and myocardial wall thickness. Martin et al. (1986) reported similar findings in trained endurance athletes, even though some training-induced adaptations were retained; there was a high positive correlation ($r > 0.80$) between left ventricular end diastolic dimension and stroke volume in all of their subjects. Despite many years of training, it takes only several weeks of detraining to induce regression of left ventricular hypertrophy. Whether training-induced adaptation of heart size and volume in highly trained athletes regresses totally with detraining is not clear (Coyle, 1998). Training-induced increase and subsequent detraining induced decrease of ventricular wall thickness, volume, and mass are independent of age up to 65 years (Giada et al., 1998).

Ventilation

Ventilatory function often parallels training-induced adaptations in $\dot{V}O_{2\,max}$. Maximum ventilatory volume declines and the ventilatory response to hypercapnia increases following long-term (2-year) detraining in highly trained athletes (Miyamura and Ishida, 1990). Short-term (10-day) detraining has no effect on ventilatory characteristics of trained distance runners, indicating that they may be protected to some extent against deterioration of ventilatory function during detraining (Cullinane et al., 1986). Ventilatory chemosensitivity is highly responsive to short-term (2-week) training in previously untrained subjects (Katayama et al., 1999).

Blood pressure

Aerobic exercise training can cause acute and chronic reduction of systolic and diastolic blood pressures with the greatest changes occurring in hypertensive persons (Fagard and Tipton, 1994). Coyle et al. (1986) found that mean blood pressure increased from 98 to 105 mmHg following 4 weeks of detraining in highly trained

Table 3.2 Metabolic adaptations to aerobic exercise training

Variables	Adaptation
Metabolic substrates	
Muscle glycogen	↑
Resting ATP	↑
Resting CP	↑
Glycolytic enzymes	
Phosphofructokinase	=
Phosphorylase	↑
Hexokinase	=
Lactate dehydrogenase	↓
Aerobic enzymes	
Citrate synthase	↑
Succinate dehydrogenase	↑
Malate dehydrogenase	↑
β-hydroxyacyl-CoA dehydrogenase	↑
Mitochondrial number/volume	↑
Lactate threshold	↑

endurance athletes; this increase was associated with a 9.4% reduction in blood volume. When blood volume was expanded to trained levels by means of infusion of dextran, however, mean blood pressure was reduced from 105 to 100 mmHg indicating that the reduction in pressure during short-term detraining is largely a result of hypovolemia. It appears that the reduced blood volume may limit ventricular filling during upright exercise, thereby compromising stroke volume and limiting cardiac output and $\dot{V}O_{2\,max}$. Thus, the reduction in stroke volume during deconditioning is largely a result of hypovolemia and not due to deterioration of heart function (Coyle, 1998).

Capillary density

Aerobic exercise training increases capillarization of the trained musculature which should enhance oxygen availability and metabolic waste removal by prolonging blood transit time and reducing diffusion distance (Coyle, 1998). Moderate training for 8 weeks elicits a 20% increase in the number of capillaries per square millimeter and per muscle fiber, and 8 weeks of detraining in these previously trained individuals results in complete reversal of those increases (Klausen et al., 1981). Similar findings have been reported by Schantz (1986) for previously untrained persons. However, Coyle et al. (1984) reported that capillarization of muscle did not change significantly following 84 days of detraining in highly trained endurance athletes; the number of capillaries per square millimeter and per muscle fiber not only remained unchanged during detraining, but were also 42% to 50% greater than sedentary controls after detraining.

Metabolic Consequences of Deconditioning

Relative to the cardiovascular consequences of deconditioning, there are relatively few data concerning the metabolic responses to deconditioning in physically active individuals. Aerobic training results in a variety of metabolic adaptations (Table 3.2) that include enhanced fat utilization, carbohydrate sparing, and reduced lactate production (Holloszy and Coyle, 1984). Increased utilization of carbohydrate during exercise after deconditioning is indicated by a higher respiratory exchange ratio during exercise (Coyle et al., 1985; Drinkwater and Horvath, 1972). Consistent with these findings is the complete reversal of epinephrine stimulated lipolysis in men and women (Despres et al., 1984) after 50 days of detraining. Hardman and Hudson (1994) also reported a reversal of a training-induced increase in high-density lipoprotein following 12 weeks of detraining. These data have been obtained from recently trained individuals; data from habitually active persons and highly trained athletes are lacking.

Carbohydrate utilization

The increased utilization of carbohydrate during detraining in highly trained individuals results in an increased blood lactate concentration during submaximal exercise at any given absolute or relative exercise intensity, and the lactate threshold occurs at a lower percentage of $\dot{V}O_{2\,max}$ following deconditioning. Following 12 weeks of detraining the lactate threshold was still higher than that of untrained controls (Coyle et al., 1985). Similar results in recently trained individuals have been reported for men (Ready and Quinney, 1982) and women (Hardman and Hudson, 1994). The increased utilization of carbohydrate following 84 days of detraining in highly trained endurance athletes is associated with increases in lactate dehydrogenase, but in little or no change in phosphofructokinase or phosphorylase (Coyle et al., 1985). One important metabolic adaptation to long-term aerobic exercise training is an increase in intracellular glycogen, whereas rapid reduction in muscle glycogen during deconditioning occurs in highly trained swimmers and in well-trained endurance athletes (Costill et al., 1985; Madsen et al., 1993).

Lipoprotein profile

Two important health benefits of aerobic exercise training are reduction in total cholesterol and an increase in the high-density lipoprotein (HDL) subfraction of total cholesterol; these responses may reduce the risk of developing cardiovascular disease (Pollock and Wilmore, 1990). Motoyama et al. (1995) observed a reversal of training-induced improvements in total and HDL cholesterol following 1 month of detraining in recently trained elderly (75-year-old) men and women. However, Cerioli et al. (1995) found no change in total or HDL cholesterol after 1 month of detraining in marathon runners.

Oxidative enzymes

In a variety of highly trained athletes there are decreases of 40% in citrate synthase, β-hydroxyacyl-CoA dehydrogenase, malate dehydrogenase, and succinate dehydrogenase activities following 4 to 12 weeks of detraining (Allen, 1989; Amigo et al., 1998; Chi et al., 1983; Coyle et al., 1984, 1985). The decline in oxidative enzyme activity during detraining occurred primarily in slow-twitch muscle fibers; fast-twitch fibers could maintain a much higher proportion of their training-induced activity. Although the influence of long-term deconditioning on mitochondrial ATP production is unknown, from the general reduction in aerobic enzyme activity it would seem that mitochondrial ATP production would be diminished as well. Indeed, Wibom et al. (1992) reported that both mitochondrial ATP production and mitochondrial enzyme activities decreased following 3 weeks of detraining in recently trained subjects.

Hormonal regulation

Hormonal regulation of metabolic activity occurs during exercise training and de-conditioning. There is little or no effect on circulating catecholamines during short-term detraining (Coyle et al., 1985; Mikines et al., 1989a;b); an exception is the reduction in insulin sensitivity (Houmard et al., 1993; Mikines et al., 1989a;b). Accompanying long-term detraining is increased catecholamine concentrations during submaximal exercise at the same absolute intensity, and reduced concentrations at the same relative intensity (Coyle et al., 1985).

Resting metabolic rate

Short-term (3-week) detraining in previously trained men does not reduce resting metabolic rate (RMR). LaForgia et al. (1999) measured the percentages of body fat and fat-free mass and RMR in eight pairs of male subjects (matched for age, body mass, and training volume) allocated to a normal training group or a detraining group. Although the detraining group showed a slight reduction in fat-free mass (0.7 kg) relative to controls, there were no significant changes in RMR following 3 weeks of detraining.

Consequences for Athletic Performance

The physiological consequences of detraining result in reduction of athletic performance. As mentioned previously, the specific health and fitness benefits from participation in physical activity are reversible, and a trained endurance athlete's performance will decline rapidly when the detraining stimulus is insufficient. Data from competitive swimmers (Claude and Sharp, 1991; Mujika et al., 1995) and distance runners (Coyle et al., 1986; Houmard et al., 1992, 1993; Madsen et al., 1993) have indicated reduction in endurance performance following detraining periods of various durations. Madsen et al. (1993) found a 21% reduction in time-to-exhaustion following just 4 weeks of detraining in well-trained endurance athletes, even though the detraining had no effect on $\dot{V}O_{2\,max}$; women exhibited reductions in both $\dot{V}O_{2\,max}$ and in time-to-exhaustion following just 2 weeks of detraining (Ready et al., 1981). These data indicate that aerobic endurance performance is rapidly compromised in both highly trained and recently trained persons. Because Ready et al.'s 1981 subjects were able to retain 24% to 38% of their training adaptation for exhaustion time and $\dot{V}O_{2\,max}$, and because Houmard et al. (1996) found no significant reduction in exercise time-to-exhaustion following 2 weeks of detraining in previously sedentary subjects, it can be presumed that performance can be maintained for up to 2 weeks during detraining.

EFFECT OF DECONDITIONING ON RESISTANCE EXERCISE TRAINING

Reduced training volume is a decrease in intensity, duration, or frequency of exercise relative to a normal level. Reasons for reducing training volume include both planned variations in training, as well as injuries and illnesses. Volume reductions are individual-specific in that a large reduction in one individual might be a small decrease or even an increase for another; for example, one person might reduce training from 5 days to 3 days per week, whereas another might reduce it from 7 days to 3 days per week. Although both are now exercising 3 days per week, the relative magnitude of reduction is different and thus the magnitude of physiological adaptation will likely be different. Clearly, the magnitude of adaptation in response to reduced training is determined by the duration and extent of detraining, with longer duration and more severe reductions in exercise leading to larger magnitude of responses.

Functional Consequences of Reduced Training

Strength

Progressive resistance exercise training increases strength, the initial improvements being chiefly a result of neural factors since changes in muscle mass may take many weeks. The most obvious functional adaptation to reduction in resistance training volume is decrease in strength that occurs regardless of testing method or type of contraction. When sedentary or recreationally active individuals must reduce their exercise volume because they have to use crutches, rapid strength losses of 0.5% to 0.6% per day occur (Adams et al., 1994; Berg et al., 1991; Hather et al., 1992a; Ploutz-Snyder et al., 1995). Alternatively, when resistance-trained athletes undergo detraining in which all formal exercise training ceases, yet maintain ambulatory function, strength losses of only 0.3% per day occur (Narici et al., 1989). These differences in strength response between sedentary and trained individuals may be determined by their initial levels of muscular fitness and the extent of exercise reduction.

Even after 8–12 weeks of detraining, athletes still maintain greater strength when compared with their pre-training status (Hakkinen et al., 1985; Hakkinen and Komi, 1983b, 1985a, 1985b; Houston et al., 1983). Detrained strength levels tend to be higher than pre-trained levels, even when the training and detraining periods are similar in length, suggesting that increases may occur more rapidly than decreases in strength. It is important to note that strength levels are retained above pre-training levels even after long periods of detraining. Staron et al. (1991) have shown that 20 weeks of resistance training in women resulted in increases of 67% to 148% in strength (depending on the exercise) and, following 30 to 32 weeks of detraining, their strength was still significantly higher than pre-training values. However, there were significant decreases in one-repetition maximum strength in the leg press (−32%) and knee extension (−29%), but not in squat exercise (−13%) when detrained values were compared with post-training values. This suggests that detraining strength decrements are not consistent in all muscle groups and exercise types. The rate of strength loss varies by muscle group and length and type of prior training. For example, training with only concentric contractions results in a more rapid detraining effect when compared with normal concentric/eccentric training, even when training volume is controlled (Colliander and Tesch, 1992; Dudley et al., 1991). However, training with only eccentric contractions results in a normal or even slower than normal detraining effect, at least over 8 weeks (Housh et al., 1996).

The findings discussed thus far relate to cessation of resistance training. There are few data on the effects of reduced training volume on muscular strength; available data indicate that strength can be maintained following training by reducing the frequency of exercise to only one session per week as long as intensity and duration are maintained (Berger, 1962; Graves et al., 1998; Hakkinen et al., 1990). It has even been suggested that the frequency can be reduced to one session every 2 or 4 weeks with minimal effect on strength, at least on lumbar muscles (Tucci et al., 1992).

Power

Power is force × velocity; therefore, to achieve high muscular power one must exert high force or high velocity. Resistance training induces an increase in muscle power, but strength decreases with detraining. If vertical jump or jump-squat performance is a gross measure of power, then changes in jump performance should mirror changes in strength. After 12 weeks of detraining following resistance training, vertical jump performance was approximately equal to pre-training levels (Hakkinen and Komi, 1985a). However, after stretch-shortening cycle training, vertical jump performance was increased by 10% above pre-training levels even after 12 weeks of detraining (Hakkinen and Komi, 1985a). There is some evidence that power declines more quickly than strength with detraining; collegiate swimmers showed no decline in shoulder strength following 4 weeks of detraining, but had an 8% to 14% decline in swimming power during the same detraining period (Wilmore and Costill, 1988).

Vulnerability to delayed-onset muscle soreness

Performance of high-intensity, different, or unusual eccentric muscle contraction causes delayed-onset muscle soreness, microscopic tissue damage, and muscle dysfunction. Recreationally active individuals are especially vulnerable to delayed-onset muscle soreness following 5 weeks of muscle unloading caused by using crutches (Ploutz-Snyder et al., 1996). Maximal eccentric contractions are usually required to induce delayed-onset muscle soreness; however, even submaximal eccentric contraction can induce muscle soreness following a period of unloading. It is possible that this soreness would be observed, to a lesser extent, in strength-trained athletes who have undergone long detraining periods. Concentric-resistance exercise training without an eccentric component renders individuals more vulnerable to delayed-onset muscle soreness and dysfunction when compared with no training (Ploutz-Snyder et al., 1998; Whitehead et al., 1998). Therefore, athletes who are performing only concentric exercise training, which is common during rehabilitation, are at greater risk of muscle soreness and dysfunction following the detraining-rehabilitation program. For this reason it is critical that rehabilitation programs include an eccentric exercise component, regardless of the training status of the individual.

Physiological Consequences of Reduced Training

Functional adaptations to reduced training are induced by morphological and physiological changes that occur in skeletal muscle with reduced use. The strength loss can be explained both by muscle fiber atrophy and associated neural changes related to recruitment of muscle fibers. Velocity and power adaptations may be induced by changes in enzyme and mitochondrial concentrations, and by changes in capillary density. From an athletic performance perspective it is easy to view decreases in strength and power as negative factors or maladaptations. However, from a physiologic perspective the decline in strength and power with disuse or reduced training are perfectly normal physiological responses. Muscle is a metabolically expensive tissue and the body is well suited to rapidly adjust the quantity and quality of muscle to match the demand placed upon it.

Muscle atrophy

Resistance exercise training induces increases in muscle size, both in single fibers and in whole muscle. Conversely, detraining induces muscle atrophy which is a reduction in skeletal muscle size. Decreases in strength are usually accompanied by muscle fiber atrophy (Hakkinen et al., 1981, 1985; Hortobagyi et al., 1993). There is some evidence that type II muscle fibers atrophy more quickly than type I fibers when there is detraining in strength-trained individuals (Hakkinen et al., 1981; Hather et al., 1992a; Staron et al., 1991) because many strength training programs induce marked type II fiber hypertrophy. Changes in muscle fiber types, particularly for short-term detraining periods, are unclear because there is little atrophy and the muscle biopsy and fiber-area measurement techniques have a variability of $\pm 10\%$.

Neural changes

Resistance training induces neural changes that rapidly facilitate force output. Increases in strength and integrated electromyographic (iEMG) activity at maximal voluntary contraction are commonly observed following training and can be reversed with detraining. Generally, maximal iEMG decreases as strength declines during detraining periods (Hakkinen et al., 1985; Hakkinen and Komi, 1983a; Houston et al., 1983; Narici et al., 1989). These neural responses represent changes in motor unit firing rate and synchronization and occur early in training/detraining programs.

Capillary density

Capillary density after training and detraining, using either concentric exercise only or a combination of concentric plus eccentric exercise training (Dudley et al., 1991; Hather et al., 1992b), indicates that both forms of training increase the number of capillaries per muscle fiber (capillary density) and that the increase can be maintained above pre-training levels throughout 4 weeks of detraining. Concentric-only training increases the number of capillaries per cross-sectional area of muscle, and this increase can be maintained during 4 weeks of detraining. This finding was a result of attenuated muscle hypertrophy and increased capillary density with concentric-only training compared with normal concentric-plus-eccentric training.

Body composition

Although muscle atrophy occurs following detraining, it is not associated with changes in percentage of body fat (Hakkinen et al., 1981, 1985; Hortobagyi et al.,

1993; Staron et al., 1991) because the variability in the measurement of lean-body mass and body-fat content is greater than the magnitude of the atrophy.

Insulin sensitivity

Strength-trained individuals have a greater physiologic response to a given amount of insulin (insulin sensitivity) than their sedentary counterparts (Fujitani et al., 1998). Resistance training itself increases whole-body insulin sensitivity in vulnerable populations such as the elderly, the glucose intolerant, and the diabetic (Eriksson et al., 1998; Miller et al., 1994; Ryan et al., 1996). Furthermore, strength training is associated with increases in glucose transporter (GLUT-4) activity and whole-body insulin sensitivity (measured with an oral glucose tolerance test). After 14 days of detraining whole-body insulin sensitivity was reduced significantly, but GLUT-4 content was maintained at 100% of the post-training content (Houmard et al., 1993). The mechanism for the detraining-induced decrease in insulin sensitivity is unclear. Dolkas and Greenleaf (1977) suggested that 1,020 kcal/day of exercise is necessary to offset hyperinsulinemia induced by bed-rest deconditioning. Those people at risk for glucose intolerance (the aged, pregnant, diabetic) should be aware that even short periods of detraining could influence their glucose tolerance and insulin sensitivity.

Hormone responses

Short periods of detraining have not been associated with marked changes in hormone activity that may be relevant for skeletal muscle function. For example, plasma concentrations of follicle-stimulating hormone, leuteinizing hormone, progesterone, estradiol, and testosterone are unchanged with short-term detraining (Hakkinen, 1989; Hakkinen and Pakarinen, 1991; Hakkinen et al., 1985, 1990). After longer-term (>12 weeks) detraining, decreases in plasma testosterone-cortisol and testosterone-sex-hormone-binding globulin ratios parallel decreases in strength (Hakkinen et al., 1985). An increase in plasma testosterone facilitates muscle hypertrophy and a decrease accompanies atrophy.

Consequences for Athletic Performance

The magnitude and extent of reduction in exercise training intensity or duration will have an important effect on athletic and work performance. The most severe reductions in training occur when trained people immobilized on crutches, by casts, or by confinement to bed rest for extended periods of time lose significant muscle mass and strength which can take months to recover (see Chapter 8 by Greenleaf). A less severe situation is that of highly trained people who discontinue exercise for an extended time and suffer large decrements in strength and power which will translate into reduced work performance. A more common deconditioning situation is that associated with seasonal variation in training, such as happens when athletes discontinue training for the summer. A recent study of adolescent soccer players reported increases in muscle enzymes and fiber area over an 11-month training period, followed by decreases after a summer (8-week) detraining period (Amigo *et al.*, 1998). The decreases were in muscle fiber cross-sectional area of Type I and Type II fibers, and in activities of creatine kinase, citrate synthase, phospho-fructokinase, lactate dehydrogenase, and aspartate aminotransferase. However, moderate detraining can also have positive effects. Many athletes begin training for their sport with intense exercise; then, as the season progresses, the training emphasis shifts from physical training to skill acquisition and practice that employ tapering-off strategies. But as long as the exercise intensity is maintained, a muscle requires only minimal stimulus to maintain strength and power. Thus, such tapering-off periods are not necessarily detrimental for performance; small decreases in strength have been documented when resistance training programs were discontinued with no detrimental effects on performance (Hoffman et al., 1991; Koutedakis, 1995; Koutedakis et al., 1992).

Reduced volume or intensity of a training program can occur because of injury, illness, or purposely before major competitions; a common practice among swimmers and some track athletes. The tapering-off protocols of these athletes usually include a period of overtraining early in the season followed by a period of reduced activity before competition. The period of reduced activity is often associated with an even increased *intensity* but with substantially reduced *duration* and *frequency* of exercise. Most types of physical performance can be maintained for weeks if intensity of training is maintained. Indeed, in people who are overtrained or tired, this approach can be quite beneficial.

EXERCISE PRESCRIPTION FOR INJURED PHYSICALLY ACTIVE INDIVIDUALS

Specific rehabilitation protocols are beyond the scope of this chapter, but several factors will be discussed. Although a period of rest or detraining may negatively affect performance in the short-term, physical injury engenders loss of short-term performance. Rehabilitation from an injury does not often require complete cessation of training, but rather a modification of training such as the water fitness and running programs often used by injured track athletes. The "unloading" effect of an aquatic environment permits some rehabilitative exercise without excessive gravitational loading on vulnerable joints. More severe injuries such as those requiring surgery, bed rest, or complete disuse of a limb will result in more substantial levels of detraining and will usually require longer periods of rehabilitation. Following periods of disuse, such as being on crutches for several weeks, skeletal muscle is particularly vulnerable to injury from eccentric exercise overload. Therefore, exercise rehabilitation treatments must progress gradually to avoid reinjury, and eccentric exercise should be an integral part of the rehabilitation program because training with only concentric contractions also produces vulnerability to injury from eccentric contractions. When applying both aerobic and anaerobic exercise during rehabilitation there is, therefore, a fine balance between providing an adequate training stimulus and avoiding reinjury.

SUMMARY

There are many health benefits associated with regular exercise training including disease prevention, management of existing disease conditions, enhanced performance of everyday activities and athletics, and improved psychosocial status. It follows that these benefits will likely be attenuated upon cessation of exercise. Few data are available on the time-course of the loss of health benefits that occur with detraining, for virtually all research on detraining has focused on physiological and performance responses. These data generally show that the time-course and severity of loss depend on the extent of detraining and the physiological systems involved. Well-documented physiological responses to detraining include decreases in $\dot{V}O_{2\,max}$, ventilatory function, lactate threshold, capillary density, muscle enzyme content, muscle strength, power, mass and performance. Detraining causes increases in heart rate, blood pressure, vulnerability to delayed-onset muscle soreness, and hyperinsulinemia. These responses may be minimized by continuing some level of physical activity, especially if exercise intensity can be maintained.

REFERENCES

Adams, G. R., Hather, B. M., and Dudley, G. A. (1994) Effect of short-term unweighting on human skeletal muscle strength and size. *Aviat. Space Environ. Med.* **65**: 1116–1121.

Allen, G. (1989) Physiological and metabolic changes with six weeks detraining. *Aust. J. Sci. Med. Sport.* **21**: 4–9.

American College of Sports Medicine (1998) ACSM Position stand on the recommended quantity and quality of exercise for developing and maintaining cardiorespiratory and muscular fitness, and flexibility in adults. *Med. Sci. Sports Exerc.* **30**: 975–991.

Amigo, N., Cadefau, J. A., Tarrados, N., and Cusso, R. (1998) Effect of summer intermission on skeletal muscle of adolescent soccer players. *J. Sports Med. Phys. Fitness* **38**: 298–304.

Barnard, R. J., Edgerton, V. R., and Peter, J. B. (1970) Effect of exercise of skeletal muscle. I. Biochemical and histochemical properties. *J. Appl. Physiol.* **28**: 762–766.

Berg, H. E., Dudley, G. A., Haggmark, T., Ohlsen, H., and Tesch, P. A. (1991) Effects of lower limb unloading on skeletal muscle mass and function in humans. *J. Appl. Physiol.* **70**: 1882–1885.

Berger, R. (1962) Effect of varied weight training programs on strength. *Res. Q. Exerc. Sport* **33**: 168–81.

Cerioli, G., Tirelli, F., and Bonetti, A. (1995) Lipoprotein (a): effect of detraining. *Acta Biomed. Ateneo Parmense* **66**: 161–167.

Chi, M.M.-Y., Hintz, C. S., Coyle, E. F., Martin, W. H., III, Ivy, J. L., Nemeth, P. M., Holloszy, J. O., and Lowry, O. H. (1983) Effects of detraining on enzymes of energy metabolism in individual human muscle fibers. *Am. J. Physiol. Cell. Physiol.* **244**: C276–C287.

Claude, A. B., and Sharp, L. B. (1991) The effectiveness of cycle ergometer training in maintaining aerobic fitness during detraining from competitive swimming. *J. Swim. Res.* **7**: 17–20.

Colliander, E., and Tesch, P. (1992) Effects of detraining following short term resistance training on eccentric and concentric muscle strength. *Acta Physiol. Scand.* **144**: 23–29.

Costill, D. L., King, D. S., Thomas, R., and Hargreaves, M. (1985) Effects of reduced training on muscular power in swimmers. *Physician Sportsmed.* **12**: 94–101.

Coyle, E. F. (1998) Deconditioning and retention of adaptations induced by endurance training. In *ACSM Resource Manual for Guidelines for Exercise Testing and Prescription*, 3rd ed. Williams & Wilkins: Baltimore, MD, pp. 189–194.

Coyle, E. F., Hemmert, M. K., and Coggan, A. R. (1986) Effects of detraining on cardiovascular responses to exercise: role of blood volume. *J. Appl. Physiol.* **60**: 95–99.

Coyle, E. G., Martin, W. H., Bloomfield, S. A., Lowry, O. H., and Holloszy, J. O. (1985) Effects of detraining on responses to submaximal exercise. *J. Appl. Physiol.* **59**: 853–859.

Coyle, E. G., Martin, W. H., Sinacore, D. R., Joyner, M. J., Hagberg, J. M., and Holloszy, J. O. (1984) Time course of loss of adaptations after stopping prolonged intense endurance training. *J. Appl. Physiol.* **57**: 1857–1864.

Cullinane, E. M., Sady, S. P., Vadeboncoeur, L., Burke, M., and Thompson, P. D. (1986) Cardiac size and $\dot{V}O_{2max}$ do not decrease after short-term exercise cessation. *Med. Sci. Sports Exerc.* **18**: 420–424.

Despres, J. P., Bouchard, C., Savard, R., Tremblay, A. Marcotte, M., and Theriault, G. (1984) Effects of exercise training and detraining on fat cell lipolysis in men and women. *Eur. J. Appl. Physiol. Occup. Physiol.* **53**: 25–30.

Dolkas, C., and Greenleaf, J. E. (1977) Insulin and glucose responses during bed rest with isotonic and isometric exercise. *J. Appl. Physiol.* **43**: 1033–1038.

Drinkwater, B., and Horvath, S. (1972) Detraining effects on young women. *Med. Sci. Sports Exerc.* **2**: 91–95.

Dudley, G. A., Tesch, P. A., Miller, B. J., and Buchanan, P. (1991) Importance of eccentric actions in performance adaptations to resistance training. *Aviat. Space Environ. Med.* **62**: 543–550.

Ehsani, A. A., Hagberg, J. M., and Hickson, R. C. (1978) Rapid changes in left ventricular dimensions and mass in response to physical conditioning and deconditioning. *Am. J. Cardiol.* **42**: 52–56.

Eriksson, J., Tuominen, J., Valle, T., Sundberg, S., Sovijarvi, A., Lindholm, H., Tuomilehto, J., and Koivisto, V. (1998) Aerobic endurance exercise or circuit-type resistance training for individuals with impaired glucose tolerance? *Horm. Metab. Res.* **30**: 37–41.

Fagard, R. H., and Tipton, C. M. (1994) Physical activity, fitness, and hypertension. In *Physical Activity, Fitness, and Health: International Proceeding and Consensus Statement*, edited by C. Bouchard, R. J. Shepard and T. Stephens, Human Kinetics: Champaign, IL, pp. 633–655.

Fournier, M., Ricci, J., Taylor, A., Gerguson, R. J., Montpeht, R. R., and Chaitman, B. R. (1982) Skeletal muscle adaptation in adolescent boys: sprint and endurance training and detraining. *Med. Sci. Sports Exerc.* **14**: 453–456.

Fringer, M. N., and Stull, G. A. (1974) Changes in cardiorespiratory parameters during periods of training and detraining in young adult females. *Med. Sci. Sports Exerc.* **6**: 20–25.

Fujitan, J., Higaki, Y., Kagawa, T., Sakamoto, M., Kiyonage, A., Shindo, M., Taniguchi, A., Nakai, Y., Tokuyama, K., and Tanaka, H. (1998) Intravenous glucose tolerance test-derived glucose effectiveness in strength-trained humans. *Metabolism* **47**: 874–877.

Giada, F., Bertaglia, E., De Picolli, B., Franceschi, M., Sartori, F., Raviele, A., and Pascotto, P. (1998) Cardiovascular adaptations to endurance training and detraining in young and older athletes. *Int. J. Cardiol.* **65**: 149–155.

Graves, J. E., Pollock, M. L., and Bryant, C. (1998) Health and fitness assessment: muscular strength and endurance. In *American College of Sports Medicine Resource Manual for Guidelines for Exercise Testing and Prescription*. Williams & Wilkins: Baltimore, MD, pp. 448–455.

Greenleaf, J. E. (1997) Intensive exercise training during bed-rest attenuates deconditioning. *Med. Sci. Sports Exerc.* **29**: 207–215.

Greenleaf, J., Jackson, C., and Lawless, D. (1994) Immune response and function: exercise conditioning versus bed-rest and spaceflight deconditioning. *Sports Med. Trng. Rehabil.* **5**: 223–241.

Hakkinen, K. (1989) Neuromuscular and hormonal adaptations during strength and power training. *Med. Sci. Sports Exerc.* **29**: 9–26.

Hakkinen, K., Alen, M., and Komi, P. V. (1985) Changes in isometric force and relaxation-time, electomyographic and muscle fibre characteristics of human skeletal muscle during strength training and detraining. *Acta Physiol. Scand.* **125**: 573–585.

Hakkinen, K., and Komi, P. V. (1983a) Changes in neuromuscular performance in voluntary and reflex contraction during strength training in man. *Int. J. Sports Med.* **4**: 282–288.

Hakkinen, K., and Komi, P. V. (1983b) Electromyographic changes during strength training and detraining. *Med. Sci. Sports Exerc.* **15**: 455–60.

Hakkinen, K., and Komi, P. V. (1985a) Changes in electrical and mechanical behavior of leg extensor muscles during heavy resistance strength training. *Scand. J. Sport Sci.* **7**: 55–64.

Hakkinen, K., and Komi, P. V. (1985b) Effect of explosive type strength training on electromyographic and force production characteristics of leg extensor muscles during concentric and various stretch-shortening cycle exercises. *Scand. J. Sport Sci.* **7**: 65–76.

Hakkinen, K., Komi, P. V., and Tesch, P. A. (1981) Effect of combined concentric and eccentric strength training and detraining on force-time, muscle fiber and metabolic characteristics of leg extensor muscles. *Scand. J. Sport Sci.* **3**: 50–58.

Hakkinen, K., and Pakarinen, A. (1991) Serum hormones in male strength athletes during intensive short term strength training. *Eur. J. Appl. Physiol.* **63**: 194–199.

Hakkinen, K., Pakarinen, A., Alen, M., and Komi, P. V. (1985) Serum hormones during prolonged training of neuromuscular performance. *Eur. J. Appl. Physiol.* **53**: 287–293.

Hakkinen, K., Pakarinen, A., Kyrolainen, H., Cheng, S., Kim, D. H., and Komi, P. V. (1990) Neuromuscular adaptations and serum hormones in females during prolonged training. *Int. J. Sports Med.* **11**: 91–98.

Hardman, A. E., and Hudson, A. (1994) Brisk walking and serum lipid and lipoprotein variables in previously sedentary women – effect of 12 weeks of regular brisk walking followed by 12 weeks of detraining. *Br. J. Sports Med.* **28**: 261–266.

Hather, B. M., Adams, G. R., Tesch. P. A., and Dudley, G.A. (1992a) Skeletal muscle responses to lower limb suspension in humans. *J. Appl. Physiol.* **72**: 1493–1498.

Hather, B., Tesch, P. A., Buchanan, P., and Dudley, G.A. (1992b) Influence of eccentric actions on skeletal muscle adaptations to resistance training. *Acta Physiol. Scand.* **143**: 177–85.

Hickson, R. C., Foster, C., Pollock, M. L., Galassi, T. M., and Rich, S. (1985) Reduced training intensities and loss of aerobic power, endurance, and cardiac growth. *J. Appl. Physiol.* **58**: 492–499.

Hickson, R. C., Kanakis, C., Jr., Davis, J. R., Moore, A. M., and Rich, S. (1982) Reduced training duration effects on aerobic power, endurance, and cardiac growth. *J. Appl. Physiol.* **53**: 225–229.

Hickson, R. C., and Rosenkoetter, M. A. (1981) Reduced training frequencies and maintenance of increased aerobic power. *Med. Sci. Sports Exerc.* **13**: 13–16.

Hoffman, J., Fray, A., Howard, R., Maresh, C. M., and Kraemer, W. J. (1991) Strength, speed, and endurance changes during the course of a Division I basketball season. *J. Appl. Sport Sci. Res.* **5**: 144–149.

Holloszy, J. O., and Coyle, E. F. (1984) Adaptations of skeletal muscle to endurance exercise and their metabolic consequences. *J. Appl. Physiol.* **56**: 831–838.

Hortobagyi, T., Houmard, J. A., Stevenson, J. R., Fraser, D. D, Johns, R. A., and Israel, R. G. (1993) The effects of detraining on power athletes. *Med. Sci. Sports Exerc.* **25**: 929–935.

Houmard, J. A., Hortobagyi, T., Johns, R. A., Bruno, N. J., Nute, C. C., Shinebarger, M. H., and Wellborn, J. W. (1992) Effect of short-term training cessation on performance measures in distance runners. *Int. J. Sports Med.* **13**: 572–576.

Houmard, J. A., Hortobagyi, T., Neufer, P. D., Johns, R. A., Fraser, D. D., and Israel, R. G. (1993) Training cessation does not alter GLUT-4 protein levels in human skeletal muscle. *J. Appl. Physiol.* **74**: 776–781.

Houmard, J. A., Tyndall, G. L., Midyette, J. B., Hickey, M. S., Dolan, P. L., Gavigan, K. E., Weidner, M. L., and Dohm, G. L. (1996) Effect of reduced training and training cessation on insulin action and muscle GLUT-4. *J. Appl. Physiol.* **81**: 1162–1168.

Housh, T., Housh, D. J., Weir, J. P., and Weir, L. L. (1996) Effects of eccentric-only resistance training and detraining. *Int. J. Sports Med.* **17**: 145–148.

Houston, M. E., Fooese, E. A., Valeriote, S. P., Green, H. G., and Ramey, D.A. (1983) Muscle performance, morphology and metabolic capacity during strength training and detraining: a one leg model. *Eur. J. Appl. Physiol.* **51**: 25–35.

Katayama, K., Sato, Y., Morotome, Y., Shima, N., Ishida, K., Mori, S., and Miyamura, M. (1999) Ventilatory chemosensitive adaptations to intermittent hypoxic exposure with endurance training and detraining. *J. Appl. Physiol.* **86**: 1805–1811.

Kiessling, K. (1971) Effects of physical training on ultrastructural features in human skeletal muscle. In *Muscle Metabolism during Exercise*, edited by B. Pernow and B. Saltin, Plenum Press: New York.

Klausen, K., Andersen, L. B., and Pelle, I. (1981) Adaptive changes in work capacity, skeletal muscle capillarization and enzyme levels during training and detraining. *Acta Physiol. Scand.* **113**: 9–16.

Koutedakis, Y. (1995) Seasonal variation in fitness parameters in competitive athletes. *Sports Med.* **19**: 373–392.

Koutedakis, Y., Boreham, C., Kabitsis, C., and Sharp, N. C. (1992) Seasonal deterioration of selected physiological variables in elite male skiers. *Int. J. Sports Med.* **13**: 548–551.

LaForgia, J., Withers, R. T., Williams, A. D., Murch, B. J., Chatterton, B. E., Schultz, C. G., and Leney, F. (1999) Effect of 3 weeks of detraining on the resting metabolic rate and body composition of trained males. *Eur. J. Clin. Nutr.* **53**: 126–133.

Madsen, K., Pedersen, P. K., Djurhuus, M. S, and Klitgaard, N. A. (1993) Effects of detraining on endurance capacity and metabolic changes during prolonged exhaustive exercise. *J. Appl. Physiol.* **75**: 1444–1451.

Martin, W. H., Coyle, E. F., Bloomfield, S. A., and Ehsani, A. A. (1986) Effects of physical deconditioning after intense endurance training on left ventricular dimensions and stroke volume. *J. Am. Coll. Cardiol.* **7**: 982–989.

McArdle, W., Katch, F., and Katch, V. (1991) *Exercise Physiology: Energy, Nutrition, and Human Performance.* Lea and Febiger: Philadelphia, PA.

Michael, E., Evert, J., and Jeffers, K. (1972) Physiological changes of teenage girls during five months of detraining. *Med. Sci. Sports* **4**: 214–218.

Mikines, K. J., Sonne, B., Tronier, B., and Galbo, H. (1989a) Effects of acute exercise and detraining on insulin action in trained men. *J. Appl. Physiol.* **66**: 704–711.

Mikines, K. J., Sonne, B., Tronier, B., and Galbo, H. (1989b) Effects of training and detraining on dose-response relationship between glucose and insulin secretion. *Am. J. Physiol. Endocrinol. Metab.* **256**: E588–E596.

Miller, J., Pratley, R. E., Goldberg, A. P., Gordon, P., Rubin, M., Treuth, M. S., Ryan, A. S., and Hurley, B. F. (1994) Strength training increases insulin action in healthy 50- to 65-yr-old men. *J. Appl. Physiol.* **77**: 1122–1127.

Miyamura, M., and Ishida, K. (1990) Adaptive changes in hypercapnic ventilatory response during training and detraining. *Eur. J. Appl. Physiol.* **60**: 353–359.

Miyashita, M., Haga, S., and Mizura, T. (1978) Training and detraining effects on aerobic power in middle-aged and older men. *J. Sports Med.* **18**: 131–137.

Moore, R. L., Thacker, E. M., Kelley, G. A., Musch, T. I., Sinoway, L.I., Foster, V.L., and Dickinson, A.L. (1987) Effect of training/detraining on submaximal exercise responses in humans. *J. Appl. Physiol.* **63**: 1719–1724.

Motoyama, M., Sunami, Y., Kinoshita, F., Irie, T., Saski, J., Arakawa, K., Kiyonaga, A., Tanaka, H., Shindo, M. (1995) The effects of long-term low intensity aerobic training and detraining on serum lipid and lipoprotein concentrations in elderly men and women. *Eur. J. Appl. Physiol.* **70**: 126–131.

Mujika, I., Chatard, J-C, Busso, T., Goyssant, A., Brale, F., and Lacoste, L. (1995) Effects of training on performance in competitive swimming. *Can. J. Appl. Physiol.* **20**: 395–406.

Narici, M. V., Roi, G. S., Landoni, L., Minetti, A. E., and Cerretelli, P. (1989) Changes in force, cross-sectional area and neural activation during strength training and detraining of the human quadriceps. *Eur. J. Appl. Physiol.* **59**: 310–319.

Neufer, P. D. (1989) The effect of detraining and reduced training on the physiological adaptations to aerobic exercise training. *Sports Med.* **8**: 302–321.

Pattengale, P. K., and Holloszy, J.O. (1967) Augmentation of skeletal muscle myoglobin by programs of treadmill running. *Am. J. Physiol.* **213**: 783–785.

Ploutz-Snyder, L. L., Tesch, P. A, Crittenden, D. J., and Dudley, G. A. (1995) Effect of unweighting on skeletal muscle use during exercise. *J. Appl. Physiol.* **79**: 168–175.

Ploutz-Snyder, L. L., Tesch, P. A., and Dudley, G. A. (1998) Increased vulnerability to eccentric exercise-induced dysfunction and muscle injury after concentric training. *Arch. Phys. Med. Rehabil.* **79**: 58–61.

Ploutz-Snyder, L. L., Tesch, P. A., Hather, B. M., and Dudley, G. A. (1996) Vulnerability to dysfunction and muscle injury after unloading. *Arch. Phys. Med. Rehabil.* **77**: 773–777.

Pollock, M. L., Mengelkoch, L. J., Graves, J. E., Lowenthal, D. T., Limacher, M. C., Foster, C., and Wilmore, J. H. (1997) Twenty-year follow-up of aerobic power and body composition of older track athletes. *J. Appl. Physiol.* **82**: 1508–1516.

Pollock, M. L., and Wilmore, J. H. (1990) *Exercise in Health and Disease*, 2nd ed. W. B. Saunders Co: Philadelphia, PA.

Ready, A. E., Eynon, R. B., and Cunningham, D. A. (1981) Effect of interval training and detraining on anaerobic fitness in women. *Can. J. Appl. Sport Sci.* **6**: 114–118.

Ready, A. E., and Quinney, H. A. (1982) Alterations in anaerobic threshold as the result of endurance training and detraining. *Med. Sci. Sports Exerc.* **14**: 292–296.

Ryan, A., Pratley, R., Goldberg, A., and Elahi, D. (1996) Resistive training increases insulin action in postmenopausal women. *J. Geront. A Biol. Sci. Med. Sci.* **51**: M199–205.

Saltin, B. (1969) Physiological effects of physical conditioning. *Med. Sci. Sports* **1**: 50–56.

Schantz, P. G. (1986) Plasticity of human skeletal muscle with specific reference to effects of physical training on enzyme levels of the NADH shuttles and phenotypic expression of slow and fast myofibrillar proteins. *Acta Physiol. Scand.* **558**: 1–62.

Simoneau, J.-A., Lortie, G., Boulay, M. R., Marcotte, M., Thibault, M. C., and Bouchard, C. (1987) Effects of two high-intensity intermittent training programs interspaced by detraining on human skeletal muscle and performance. *Eur. J. Appl. Physiol.* **56**: 516–521.

Staron, R. S., Leonardi, M. J., Karapondo, D. L., Malicky, E. S., Falkel, J. E., Hagerman, F. C., and Hikida, R. S. (1991) Strength and skeletal muscle adaptations in heavy-resistance-trained women after detraining and retraining. *J. Appl. Physiol.* **70**: 631–640.

Tucci, J. T., Carpenter, D. M., Pollock, M. L., Graves, J. E., and Leggett, S.H. (1992) Effect of reduced frequency of training and detraining on lumbar extension strength. *Spine* **17**: 1497–1501.

U.S. Department of Health and Human Services (1996) Physical Activity and Health: A report of the Surgeon General. Centers for Disease Control and Prevention, National Center for Chronic Disease Prevention and Health Promotion, Atlanta, GA.

Wang, J.-S., Jen, C. J., Chen, H.-I. (1997) Effects of chronic exercise and deconditioning on platelet function in women. *J. Appl. Physiol.* **83**: 2080–2085.

Whitehead, N. P., Allen, T. J., Morgan, D. L., and Proske, U. (1998) Damage to human muscle from eccentric exercise after training with concentric exercise. *J. Physiol. (Lond.)* **15**: 615–620.

Wibom, R. E., Hultman, E., Johansson, M., Matherei, K., Constantin-Teodosiu, D., and Schantz, P. G. (1992) Adaptation of mitochondrial ATP production in human skeletal muscle to endurance training and detraining. *J. Appl. Physiol.* **73**: 2004–2010.

Wilmore, J. H., Costill, D. L. (1988) *Training for Sport and Activity, The Physiological Basis of the Conditioning Process*, 3rd ed., Human Kinetics: Champaign, IL.

CHAPTER 4

Immobilization and Disuse Muscular Atrophy

Shawn R. Simonson

Department of Wellness and Movement Sciences,
Western New Mexico University, Silver City, New Mexico, USA

> Under the spreading chestnut tree
> The village smithy stands;
> The smith, a mighty man is he,
> With large and sinewy hands;
> And the muscles of his brawny arms
> Are strong as iron bands...
> He earns whate'er he can,
> And looks the whole world in the face,
> For he owes not any man.
>
> *Henry Wadsworth Longfellow*

INTRODUCTION

The reduction or cessation of physical training or of normal ambulatory exertions that result from prolonged bed rest or from the immobilization of healthy or injured limbs produce significant effects on the body's muscular performance. Disuse of muscles, whatever the cause of the immobilization, stimulates both local and whole-body adaptations; it is these local muscular effects that will be discussed here.

MUSCULAR ENDURANCE

Muscular endurance decreases with reduction in use of a muscle whether the result of immobilization or of a decrease in daily physical activity. Endurance is reduced

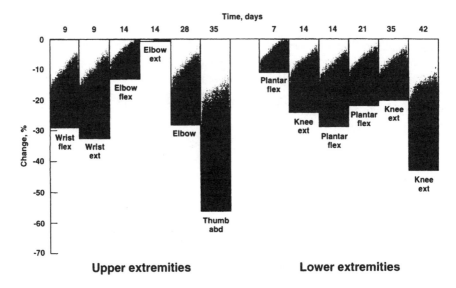

Figure 4.1   Mean percent changes in maximal muscular strength from 7 to 42 days of upper and lower extremity immobilization: ext = extension, flex = flexion. (From Davies et al., 1987; Dudley et al., 1992; Hislop, 1964; Miles et al., 1994; Ploutz-Snyder et al., 1995; Sale et al., 1982; Stillwell et al., 1967; Vaughan, 1989; White et al., 1984.)

by 27% after 31 days of postoperative immobilization (Halkjaer-Kristensen and Ingemann-Hansen, 1985b). In ambulatory persons following cessation of both endurance and strength training there is no loss of muscular endurance after 1 week; however, there is a significant loss after 3 weeks (Shaver, 1973; Sysler and Stull, 1970). Additional decrements may (Shaver, 1973) or may not (Sysler and Stull, 1970) continue to the fifth week. After 8 weeks of deconditioning, the loss of endurance levels off and does not progress further by week 12; exercise conditioning prior to limb immobilization or reduced activity provides some protection in that endurance does not deteriorate to pre-training levels after 12 weeks of deconditioning (Waldman and Stull, 1969).

PEAK TORQUE

Torque is "the degree to which a force tends to rotate an object about a specified fulcrum" (Harman, 1994). Peak torque—the peak force times the length of the moment arm that can be generated to rotate a limb about a joint—can be concentric (muscle shortening with the contraction), eccentric (muscle lengthening with the contraction), or isometric (no change in muscle length with contraction). Thirty-one days of post-injury immobilization (without surgical intervention) did not reduce concentric peak torque; however, with surgery it declined by 47% to 52%

(Halkjaer-Kristensen and Ingemann-Hansen, 1985b). Isometric peak torque can be reduced by 80% after 6 weeks of immobilization (Morrissey et al., 1985) and by 45% after 2 weeks to 7 months (Stillwell et al., 1967).

Immobilization of limbs in healthy subjects decreases peak torque. Greater decrements appear after a few days, with a gradual decay and a leveling off between 2 and 4 weeks. Concentric peak torque fell 9% to 22% (depending on the speed of movement, with greater decrements at faster speeds) after 9 days (Miles et al., 1994); it decreased 17% after 10 days (Gamrin et al., 1998), 20% after 4 weeks (Berg et al., 1991), and by only 21% after 6 weeks (Dudley et al., 1992). Eccentric peak torque appears to follow the same trend of decreasing by 12% to 19% (greater decrements at faster speeds) after 9 days (Miles et al., 1994), and by 23% after 4 weeks (Berg et al., 1991). Both initial peak torque (average of the first five contractions) and average peak torque (average of 30 contractions) fell by 17% over 4 weeks (Berg et al., 1993). Isometric peak torque declined by 12% to 28% (greater decrements at faster speeds) after 2 weeks of limb immobilization (Stillwell et al., 1967). Isometric peak torque (using a concentric contraction) decreased by 18%, and torque with an eccentric contraction fell by 15% (Berg et al., 1991). In a healthy limb the combination of injury and immobilization causes greater loss of peak torque than only immobilization.

Cessation of physical training (deconditioning) reduces peak torque, but it is neither as rapid nor as severe as that found after limb immobilization. There was no change in concentric peak torque after 4 weeks of deconditioning, but it decreased by 16% to 21% (greater decrements at faster speeds) after 12 weeks (Houston et al., 1983). On the other hand, isometric peak torque decreased by only 7% to 8% after 8 weeks of post-training deconditioning (Hakkinen and Komi, 1983).

MAXIMAL STRENGTH

Strength is the maximal force generated by muscular contraction without regard for time (one repetition maximum or a maximal voluntary contraction). It is different from peak torque in that rotation about an axis is not considered; it is just the exertion of force. Strength declines with immobilization and cessation of training.

Strength is reduced after 22 days of post-injury immobilization (Jenkins et al., 1976); at 31 days it had declined by 43 to 58% (Fuglsang-Frederiksen and Scheel, 1978; Halkjaer-Kristensen and Ingemann-Hansen, 1985b). There does not appear to be a further deterioration in strength with immobilization to 135 days (Duchateau and Hainut, 1989; Duchateau and Hainut, 1987; Fuglsang-Frederiksen and Scheel, 1978; Stillwell et al., 1967; White and Davies, 1984).

Immobilization of a healthy limb causes loss of strength, although not as great a loss as occurs in an injured limb. Immobilization appears to cause greater and faster strength losses in the upper extremities than in the lower extremities (Figure 4.1) (Davies et al., 1987; Dudley et al., 1992; Hislop, 1964; Miles et al., 1994; Ploutz-Snyder et al., 1995; Sale et al., 1982; Stillwell et al., 1967; Vaughan, 1989; White et al., 1984).

With the cessation of arm training there is little alteration in strength during the first week (Shaver, 1973; Shaver, 1975); however, a significant reduction occurs by 3 weeks and continues to 6 weeks (41%) when strength loss is attenuated; there is no additional loss to 8 weeks (MacDougall et al., 1980; Shaver, 1973, 1975). Hakkinen et al. (1981) found a smaller reduction (12%) in leg strength; thus, the upper extremities may experience greater decrements. Narici et al. (1989) calculated that strength decreased by 0.3% per day of deconditioning.

ELECTROMYOGRAPHY

Electromyographic (EMG) activity decreases during muscular contractions following both immobilization and deconditioning in both injured and healthy limbs. This decreased activity occurs within 3 days of post-injury immobilization (Wolf et al., 1971) and can reach 45% by 8 weeks (Duchateau and Hainut, 1989). After 4 to 6 weeks of post-injury immobilization, increasing the resistant force did not increase the firing frequency of the immobilized muscle as much as in the contralateral control (Fuglsang-Frederiksen and Scheel, 1978). Electromyographic activity in a healthy limb decreases by 36% after 2 weeks of immobilization (Vaughan, 1989), whereas activity at the same relative load (35% of maximum voluntary contraction) was unchanged (Fuglevand et al., 1995). However, the EMG activity during pre-determined absolute loads increased by 300% to 600% after 6 weeks of immobilization (Dudley et al., 1992).

It is clear that reductions in EMG activity during limb immobilization with and without injury are uniformly 6% to 12% greater than that following the cessation of training (Hakkinen and Komi, 1983). The rate of loss of EMG activity (with training cessation) is about 0.7% per day of disuse (Narici et al., 1989).

ELECTRICAL STIMULATION

Electrical stimulation can be used to determine whether the deconditioning was associated more with neural or local muscular factors. If the response to electrical stimulation does not change after deconditioning, then neural factors are probably the cause of performance decrements. On the other hand, if muscular alterations predominate, then there will be changes in the response to electrical stimulation.

Muscular contraction time of an injured limb increases by 13% to 16% after 6 to 8 weeks of immobilization (Duchateau and Hainut, 1989). The time required for a muscle to reach peak tension (TPT) increases by 16% after 8 weeks (Duchateau and Hainut, 1987) and decreases by 25% after 135 days of immobilization (White and Davies, 1984). The half relaxation time (1/2 RT), the time for the muscle to release half of a generated contraction, increased by 14% after 6 to 8 weeks of immobilization (Duchateau and Hainut, 1987, 1989) and does not decrease further by 135 days (White and Davies, 1984). The magnitude of the decreases in maximal twitch tetanic tension is similar to those for maximal voluntary contraction force; for example, by 33% after 6 to 8 weeks (Duchateau and Hainut, 1987, 1989) and up to 51% by 135 days (White and Davies, 1984). The fatigue index (rate of decay of mechanical tension) is unchanged by immobilization (Duchateau and Hainut, 1987, 1989).

Immobilization of a healthy limb elicited the same alteration in TPT as did an injured limb. It increased by 13% in the first week and remained unchanged after 14 days (White et al., 1984) and 21 days (Davies et al., 1987). The 1/2 RT (leg) increased by 22% in the first week, did not change in the second (White et al., 1984), and was at 18% (forearm) after 21 days (Davies et al., 1987). Maximal twitch tetanic tension was unchanged after the first week (White et al., 1984) and decreased by 10% after the third week (Davies et al., 1987), while the fatigue index was unchanged (Davies et al., 1987; Fuglevand et al., 1995; Miles et al., 1994; White et al., 1984).

The cessation of training alone did not affect the 1/2 RT after 12 weeks of deconditioning (Hakkinen et al., 1985), but the maximal twitch tetanic tension decreased by 25% after 5 weeks of deconditioning (Sale et al., 1982).

Thus, it appears that local muscle adaptation and not neural factors is primarily responsible for the loss of function resulting from immobilization or cessation of training.

BLOOD AND MUSCLE BIOCHEMISTRY

The blood acid (lactate) – base (bicarbonate) relationship changes with conditioning and deconditioning (Costill et al., 1985). Resting lactate is elevated with leg immobilization (Richter et al., 1989) but unaffected by arm immobilization (Ward et al., 1986); exercise blood lactate was decreased by 23% after 2 weeks of deconditioning from running (Houston et al., 1979). In contrast, after 4 weeks of detraining blood lactate increased by 131% above the trained level in competitive swimmers (Costill et al., 1985; Neuffer et al., 1987) during a swimming challenge, but by only 5% for single arm exercise (Ward et al., 1986). This large difference in the exercise-induced increase in lactate is probably a result of the muscle mass involved. Increases in blood lactate may indicate decreases in lactate clearance, aerobic ATP generation, efficiency, or alterations in local blood flow (Costill et al., 1985; Neuffer et al., 1987; Ward et al., 1986). Decreases in blood lactate might indicate reduced aerobic capacity and anaerobic energy production, or alterations in local blood flow (Houston et al., 1979). There were no changes in blood lactate with cessation of activity by the elderly or by those participating in a low-intensity exercise program (Orlander et al., 1977; Pickering et al., 1997).

Data from the intracellular biochemical environment by means of muscle biopsy also reflect the decrease in muscle function during deconditioning. Two of three electrolytes involved in establishing the membrane potential are altered: Cl^- increases by 111%, Na^+ increases by 37%, and K^+ is unchanged; whereas, those that do not affect the membrane potential (PO_4^{3-} and S^{2-}) are unchanged (Wroblewski et al., 1987).

The energy-rich phosphates do not respond appreciably to training or detraining. ATP does not change (Gamrin et al., 1998; MacDougall et al., 1977; Ward et al., 1986) and phosphocreatine and total creatine do not change after 10 days of leg immobilization (Gamrin et al., 1998); but both decrease by 23% after 5 weeks of arm immobilization (MacDougall et al., 1977; Ward et al., 1986). However, muscle glycogen is reduced by 26% to 45% after 4 to 5 weeks of training cessation (Costill et al. 1985; MacDougall et al., 1977; Ward et al., 1986).

There is some disagreement about alterations in net intracellular protein content during immobilization and detraining because there is no change in the total amino acid concentration (Gamrin et al., 1998); but there is reduction in total protein concentration (Gibson et al., 1987). Is the latter a reduction in protein anabolism or an increase in protein catabolism, or some combination? Injury and duration of immobilization cloud this picture; for example, 10 days of immobilization of a healthy leg did not change protein synthesis (Gamrin et al., 1998), but 37 days of immobilization of an injured leg reduced anabolism by 26% (Gibson et al., 1987). Protein catabolism may also be increased (Gibson et al., 1987) resulting in a protein concentration reduced by a decrease in anabolism and an increase in catabolism (Gibson et al., 1987; Rennie et al., 1983).

Protein production during immobilization of the healthy limb causes no change in the ribosome concentration; however, the RNA content decreased by 16% during 10 days of limb immobilization (Gamrin et al., 1998). In the injured limb, 38 days of immobilization reduced RNA activity by 48% compared with the contralateral control (Gibson et al., 1987); the DNA content was unchanged (Gamrin et al., 1998).

Because alterations in intracellular and plasma amino acid concentrations respond differently, plasma concentrations are not indicative of activity within the muscle; thus, a muscle biopsy must be done to understand the local effects of immobilization (unloading) or disuse (Vinnars et al., 1975). From the few available data it seems that although muscle RNA concentration is decreased during leg unloading, protein synthesis and total amino acid concentration are unaltered (Gamrin et al., 1998): muscle asparagine, carnosine, glutamine, histidine, isoleucine, methionine, ornithine, and threonine are unchanged (Gamrin et al., 1998; Vinnars et al., 1975). Intracellular markers of protein breakdown increase; branched chain amino acids (+49%) and asparagine, citrulline, phenylalanine, and threonine (Gamrin et al., 1998; Vinnars et al., 1975). Muscle alanine, glycine, leucine, lysine, serine, taurine, tyrosine, and valine also increase while muscle arginine, glutamate, glutamine, and proline decrease (Vinnars et al., 1975).

The enzymes involved in energy transport are also affected differently by the disuse associated with immobilization or detraining. ATPase is unchanged by 5 to 6 weeks of detraining (MacDougall et al., 1980). Creatine kinase (CK) is decreased by 12% 6 weeks post-surgery; the CK MB isoform falls by 18% and the mitochondrial isoform by 4% (Jansson et al., 1987). The detraining data are ambiguous showing no change in aerobic athletes (Chi et al., 1983; Houston et al., 1983) and an increase or a decrease after resistance training (Hakkinen et al., 1981; MacDougall et al., 1977).

Hexokinase, the first enzyme in glycolysis appears to be slow to respond to cessation of aerobic training; there was no change measured after 15 days of detraining (Houston et al., 1983), but a 17% decrease after 6 to 12 weeks of detraining (Chi et al., 1983). HAD (3-hydroxyacyl CoA dehydrogenase), involved in fatty acid oxidation, exhibits the same slow responses; there is no change after 15 days (Houston et al., 1983) but a decrease of 14% by 8 weeks (Orlander et al., 1977). However, Richter et al. (1989) found a similar relative decrease in HAD after only 7 days of immobilization. Myokinase is unchanged (Hakkinen et al., 1981).

Not only energy utilization but energy substrate uptake may also be changed by disuse. Glucose uptake is reduced by 13% after 7 days of healthy leg immobilization (Richter et al., 1989); a reduction of 17% by 6 days to 33% by 10 days in the GLUT-4 transport molecule may be responsible (McCoy et al., 1994; Vukovich et al., 1996). However, no change in GLUT-4 transport was noted in either endurance- or strength-trained individuals after 14 days of training cessation (Houmard et al., 1993). Lipo-protein lipase (free fatty acid uptake molecule) activity is also reduced after 14 days of detraining (Simsolo et al., 1993).

Oxidative enzymes, thus the oxidative capacity of the muscle cell, are also reduced by disuse; this reduction is especially pronounced in the slow-twitch oxidative (SO) fibers (Haggmark et al., 1981). Aspartate aminotransferase decreases by 30% 6 weeks after post-anterior cruciate ligament (ACL) surgery immobilization (Jansson et al., 1987). Activity of β-hydroxyacyl-CoA dehydrogenase falls by 34% and activity of malate dehydrogenase declines by 29% with 6 to 12 weeks of detraining (Chi et al., 1983). NADH tetrazolium reductase is unchanged (Halkjaer-Kristensen and Ingemann-Hansen, 1985d) as is pyruvate dehydrogenase activity and concentration (Ward et al., 1986); however, pyruvate dehydrogenase responsiveness to exercise is reduced with immobilization (Ward et al., 1986). Succinate dehydrogenase activity is not affected by 14 days of detraining (Houston et al., 1983), but is reduced by 19% to 35% with 5 to 6 weeks of post-injury immobilization or with 12 weeks of detraining (Chi et al., 1983; Coyle et al., 1984; Haggmark et al., 1981; Halkjaer-Kristensen and Ingemann-Hansen, 1985d). Six to 8 weeks of detraining will return it to pre-conditioning levels (Henriksson and Reitman, 1977; Klausen et al., 1980). Reductions in succinate dehydrogenase may be preferential to SO fibers with a 53% reduction compared with a 33% decrease in fast-twitch-glycolytic (FG) and fast-twitch oxidative/glycolytic (FOG) fibers (Castro et al., 1999; Haggmark et al., 1981).

Citrate synthase decreases in injury-induced immobilization and in aerobically trained individuals who detrain: by 9% after 10 days to 400% after 84 days (Berg et al., 1993; Chi et al., 1983; Coyle et al., 1984; Houmard et al., 1992, 1993; McCoy et al., 1994; Moore et al., 1987), and the reductions are directly proportional to the duration of conditioning and inactivity (Moore et al., 1987). There does not appear to be any citrate synthase decrement in those who have ceased strength-training (Houmard et al., 1993).

Cytochrome C decreases within 2 weeks of detraining and continues to fall by weeks 4 to 6. By 6 weeks it has returned to pre-training levels and does not fall further (Henriksson and Reitman, 1977; Klausen et al., 1980). The lower levels of cytochrome C reduce the ability to oxidize free fatty acids and may be related to the decrease in lipoprotein lipase.

The glycolytic/glycogenolytic enzymes also have varied responses to immobilization and detraining. Adenylate kinase, fructose biphosphatase (Chi et al., 1983), phosphofructokinase (Berg et al., 1993; Chi et al., 1983; Costill et al., 1985; Haggmark et al., 1981; Halkjaer-Kristensen and Ingemann-Hansen, 1985d; Houston et al., 1983; Jansson et al., 1987; Klausen et al., 1980; Orlander et al., 1977), and phosphorylase (Chi et al., 1983; Costill et al., 1985) are all unaltered. However, Klausen et al. (1980) reported a reduction in phosphorylase during detraining. This difference in phosphorylase responses may have been peculiar to the populations studied; that is, inactive individuals who were trained and then detrained (Klausen et al., 1980) versus athletes detraining (Chi et al., 1983; Costill et al., 1985). Increases in α-glycerophosphate dehydrogenase occurred in both Type I and Type II muscle fibers, with Type I being the most affected in injured and immobilized individuals (Castro et al., 1999; Halkjaer-Kristensen and Ingemann-Hansen, 1985d); but it is unaltered in subjects who have ceased participation in a very low-intensity aerobic conditioning program (Orlander et al., 1977). Lactate dehydrogenase is unaltered when strength training stops (Houston et al., 1983), but decreases with cessation of aerobic training or with injury-induced immobilization (Houston et al., 1979; Jansson et al., 1987) and will return to pre-training levels by 4 weeks of inactivity (Klausen et al., 1980). However, Chi (1983) found increases in lactate dehydrogenase when endurance-trained runners ceased training for 6 to 12 weeks. Myoglobin, the muscular oxygen transport molecule, increased during injury-induced immobilization (Jansson et al., 1987) but was unaffected by 2 to 12 weeks of training cessation (Coyle et al., 1984).

Muscle fat and water contents are unchanged during immobilization of a healthy limb (Gamrin et al., 1998).

The effect of deconditioning on the number of capillaries per muscle fiber has been determined from muscle biopsies, and there is some discrepancy when immobilization data are compared with detraining data. The number of capillaries per fiber (all fiber types) is unchanged during immobilization of the healthy limb in untrained individuals (Berg et al., 1993; Hather et al., 1992). However, cessation of training causes a decrease of 11%, with the greatest loss occurring by week 4; Type I fibers decrease by 16%, Type IIa fibers by 10%, and Type IIb fibers by 14% (Klausen et al., 1980).

ATROPHY

Muscle atrophy occurs in unused limbs; circumference is reduced by 10% to 13% as a result of injury and immobilization (Haggmark et al., 1981; Lindboe and Platou, 1982; Morrissey et al., 1985; Wolf et al., 1971), by immobilization of a healthy limb, or by discontinuation of training (Hakkinen et al., 1985; 1981; Ingemann-Hansen and Halkjaer-Kristensen, 1977; MacDougall et al., 1977). Limb cross-sectional area is decreased by 2% to 5% (Miles et al., 1994; White et al., 1984) after 1 week of immobilization and by an additional 3% by week 2 (White et al., 1984). Limb volume decreases by 5% to 12% because of injury and immobilization (Davies and Sargeant, 1975; Gibson et al., 1987; Halkjaer-Kristensen and Ingemann-Hansen, 1985a; Ingemann-Hansen and Halkjaer-Kristensen, 1977; Sargeant et al., 1977) and also by 5% to 10% with immobilization alone (Hislop, 1964; Richter et al., 1989). There appears to be little difference between the effects of injury, immobilization, or disuse on muscle atrophy.

Most atrophy is the result of decrease in muscle cross-sectional area because the limb fat compartment does not appear to be affected by deconditioning (Berg et al., 1991; Halkjaer-Kristensen and Ingemann-Hansen, 1985a; Ingemann-Hansen and Halkjaer-Kristensen, 1977). In the healthy leg, immobilized cross-sectional area of the ankle extensor muscles decreased by 14% to 18% after 6 weeks (Dudley et al., 1992; Hather et al., 1992), with the gastrocnemius losing 26% and the soleus 17% (Hather et al., 1992). The total mid-thigh muscle cross-sectional area decreased by 7% to 12% in 4 to 6 weeks (Berg et al., 1991; Hather et al., 1992) at a rate of about 0.1% per day (Narici et al., 1989). The primary locomotive muscles of the thigh (quadriceps) are affected more than the hamstrings with decreases of 8% to 27% over a period of 16 days to 6 weeks (Adams et al., 1994; Dudley et al., 1992; Halkjaer-Kristensen and Ingemann-Hansen, 1985c; Hather et al., 1992; Ingemann-Hansen and Halkjaer-Kristensen, 1980; Ploutz-Snyder et al., 1995; Young et al., 1982). The hamstring group is either unaffected (Adams et al., 1994; Young et al., 1982) or decreased by 4% to 7% (Halkjaer-Kristensen and Ingemann-Hansen, 1985a; Hather et al., 1992) post-immobilization with or without injury. The forearm loses 4% of muscle cross-sectional area after 9 days of immobilization (Miles et al., 1994).

Muscle fiber size decreases by 38% in patients with knee injuries without joint immobilization (Young et al., 1982). Type I (SO) fiber size (decreased by 39%) tended to be less affected than Type II (decreased by 46%) when compared with the contralateral limb (Young et al., 1982). When an injury is accompanied by immobilization there does not appear to be a difference in fiber type atrophy after 5 days (Lindboe and Platou, 1982), but over 5 weeks of immobilization the postural endurance muscle (SO) fibers tend to atrophy more than the FG or FOG fibers (Gibson et al., 1987; Haggmark et al., 1981). The immobilization-induced atrophy within the healthy limb is not as great, nor does it occur as rapidly, for there was no change in fiber size after 4 weeks of immobilization (Adams et al., 1994; Berg et al., 1993); but by 6 weeks of unloading there was a total decrease of 14%, with Type I size decreasing by 12% and Type II by 15% (Type IIa decreased, IIb unchanged) (Hather et al., 1992). Others have found no alteration in Type II fiber cross-sectional area with training cessation (Larsson and Ansved, 1985).

When athletes decondition the cross-sectional area decreases for all fiber types, but there is little consensus as to the degree and preferential atrophy. Some have found no alteration after 2 weeks or up to 42 months of detraining by athletes (Chi et al., 1983; Houmard et al., 1992; Larsson and Ansved, 1985); others have reported that fast-twitch fibers atrophy more than slow-twitch fibers, with Type IIb fibers exhibiting the greatest loss when untrained individuals are trained and then detrained

(Hakkinen et al., 1985; Klausen et al., 1980). Thus, the degree and fiber-type atrophy are different with duration of previous training; short-term training adaptations are lost rapidly, and those after long-term training are retained longer.

FIBER NUMBER AND RELATIVE PERCENTAGE

Fiber numbers and relative percentage of fiber populations have also been determined from muscle biopsies. The 21% decrease of total muscle fiber content 31 days post-surgery is a result of a total fiber number loss of 28% (Halkjaer-Kristensen and Ingemann-Hansen, 1985c). The Type I (SO) muscle fibers are more susceptible to this atrophy with decrements of 8 to 21% over 31 to 35 days (Haggmark et al., 1981; Halkjaer-Kristensen and Ingemann-Hansen, 1985c). This predominantly type I atrophy trend does not exist after spinal cord injury that results in limb paralysis; the percent of Type I increased by 5%, while Type IIa decreased by 56%, and Type IIax + IIx increased by 36% (Castro et al., 1999). A reduction in the percentage of one fiber type must be reflected in an increased percentage of the other (Haggmark et al., 1986).

Immobilization without injury presents a different response, for there is no change in fiber type composition (no preferential atrophy) after 49 days (Adams et al., 1994; Berg et al., 1993; Hather et al., 1992).

Again, the detraining picture is not as clear. No preferential atrophy is found after a layoff of 12 weeks from strength training or 8 weeks from low-intensity aerobic conditioning (Houston et al., 1983; Orlander et al., 1977). However, there is a 14% to 25% decrease in the relative percentage of Type I fibers 8 weeks to 42 months after ceasing aerobic athletic training (Klausen et al., 1980; Larsson and Ansved, 1985) which leads to an increase in the relative percentage of Type II fibers (Klausen et al., 1980).

CONNECTIVE TISSUE

The effects of muscle immobilization or disuse on the tissues to which the muscles connect must also be considered. A complete review of this is beyond the scope of this chapter, but the connective tissues are affected, although less significantly than the muscle itself because they have a lower metabolism (Kannus et al., 1992). The muscle–tendon junction atrophies and weakens, and the contact area decreases by 16.5% in 1 week. Proprioceptive mechanisms within the muscle and muscle–tendon junction degenerate and are not as responsive. The tendon itself loses tensile strength and elastic stiffness because the collagen fibers atrophy, disorganize, and there is a decrease in cross-link number and size. Ligament total collagen mass also decreases (Kannus et al., 1992), periarticular soft tissue rigidity increases, and the joint capsule shrinks (Appell, 1990).

SUMMARY

It is apparent that there are three levels of disuse atrophy and associated reductions in performance. In order of greatest atrophy and decrement of performance they are (1) injury with immobilization, (2) immobilization of the healthy limb, and (3) cessation of training. The metabolic activity of the tissue, the degree of disuse, and the previous state of training all affect the degree of atrophy.

REFERENCES

Adams, G. R., Hather, B. M., and Dudley, G. A. (1994) Effect of short-term unweighting on human skeletal muscle strength and size. *Aviat. Space Environ. Med.* **65**: 1116–1121.

Appell, H.-J. (1990) Muscular atrophy following immobilization: a review. *Sports Med.* **10**: 42–58.

Berg, H. E., Dudley, G. A., Haggmark, T., Ohlsen, H., and Tesch, P. A. (1991) Effects of lower limb unloading on skeletal muscle mass and function in humans. *J. Appl. Physiol.* **70**: 1882–1885.

Berg, H. E., Dudley, G. A., Hather, B., and Tesch, P. A. (1993) Work capacity and metabolic and morphologic characteristics of the human quadriceps muscle in response to unloading. *Clin. Physiol.* **13**: 337–347.

Castro, M. J., Apple, D. F., Staron, R.S., Campos, G. E. R., and Dudley, G. A. (1999) Influence of complete spinal cord injury on skeletal muscle within 6 mo of injury. *J. Appl. Physiol.* **86**: 350–358.

Chi, M. M.-Y., Hintz, C. S., Coyle, E. F., Martin, W. H., III, Ivy, J. L., Nemeth, P. M., Holloszy, J. O., and Lowry, O. H. (1983) Effects of detraining on enzymes of energy metabolism in individual human muscle fibers. *Am. J. Physiol. Cell. Physiol.* **244**: C276–C287.

Costill, D. L., Fink, W. J., Hargreaves, M. , King, D. S., Thomas, R., and Fielding, R. (1985) Metabolic characteristics of skeletal muscle during detraining from competitive swimming. *Med. Sci. Sports Exerc.* **17**: 339–343.

Coyle, E. F., Martin, W. H., III, Sinacore, D. R., Joyner, M. J., Hagberg, J. M., and Holloszy, J. O. (1984) Time course of loss of adaptations after stopping prolonged intense endurance training. *J. Appl. Physiol.* **57**: 1857–1864.

Davies, C. T. M., Rutherford, I. C., and Thomas, D. O. (1987) Electrically evoked contractions of the triceps surae during and following 21 days of voluntary leg immobilization. *Eur. J. Appl. Physiol.* **56**: 306–312.

Davies, C. T. M., and Sargeant, A. J. (1975) Effects of exercise therapy on total and component tissue leg volumes of patients undergoing rehabilitation from lower limb injury. *Ann. Hum. Biol.* **2**: 327–337.

Duchateau, J., and Hainut, K. (1987) Electrical and mechanical changes in immobilized human muscle. *J. Appl. Physiol.* **62**: 2168–2173.

Duchateau, J., and Hainut, K. (1989) Effects of immobilization on contractile properties, recruitment and firing rates of human motor units. *J. Physiol.* (Lond.) **422**: 55–65.

Dudley, G. A., Duvoisin, M. R., Adams, G. R., Meyer, R. A., Belew, A. H., and Buchanan, P. (1992) Adaptations to unilateral lower limb suspension in humans. *Aviat. Space Environ. Med.* **63**: 678–683.

Fuglevand, A. J, Bilodeau, M., and Enoka, R. M. (1995) Short-term immobilization has a minimal effect on the strength and fatigability of a human hand muscle. *J. Appl. Physiol.*

78: 847–855.

Fuglsang-Frederiksen, A., and Scheel, U. (1978) Transient decrease in number of motor units after immobilization in man. *J. Neurol. Neurosurg. Psychiatry* **41**: 924–929.

Gamrin, L., Berg, H. E., Essen, P., Tesch, P. A., Hultman, E., Garlick, P. J., McNurlan, M. A., and Wernerman, J. (1998) The effect of unloading on protein synthesis in human skeletal muscle. *Acta Physiol. Scand.* **163**: 369–377.

Gibson, J. N. A., Halliday, D., Morrison, W. L., Stoward, P. J., Hornsby, G. A., Wyatt, P. W., Murdoch, G., and Rennie, M. J. (1987) Decrease in human quadriceps muscle protein turnover consequent upon leg immobilization. *Clin. Sci.* **72**: 503–509.

Haggmark, T., Eriksson, E., and Jansson, E. (1986) Muscle fiber type changes in human skeletal muscle after injuries and immobilization. *Orthopedics* **9**: 181–185.

Haggmark, T., Jansson, E., and Eriksson, E. (1981) Fiber type area and metabolic potential of the thigh muscle in man after knee surgery and immobilization. *Int. J. Sports Med.* **2**: 12–17.

Hakkinen, K., Alen, M., and Komi, P. V. (1985) Changes in isometric force- and relaxation-time, electromyographic and muscle fibre characteristics of human skeletal muscle during strength training and detraining. *Acta Physiol. Scand.* **125**: 573–585.

Hakkinen, K., and Komi, P. V. (1983) Electromyographic changes during strength training and detraining. *Med. Sci. Sports Exerc.* **15**: 455–460.

Hakkinen, K., Komi, P. V., and Tesch, P.A. (1981) Effect of combined concentric and eccentric strength training and detraining on force-time, muscle fiber and metabolic characteristics of leg extensor muscles. *Scand. J. Sports Sci.* **3**: 50–58.

Halkjaer-Kristensen, J., and Ingemann-Hansen, T. (1985a) Wasting of the human quadriceps muscle after knee ligament injuries: I, anthropometrical consequences. *Scand. J. Rehab. Med.* **13**: 5–11.

Halkjaer-Kristensen, J., and Ingemann-Hansen, T. (1985b) Wasting of the human quadriceps muscle after knee ligament injuries: IV, dynamic and static muscle function. *Scand. J. Rehab. Med.* **13**: 29–37.

Halkjaer-Kristensen, J., and Ingemann-Hansen, T. (1985c) Wasting of the human quadriceps muscle after knee ligament injuries: II, muscle fiber morphology. *Scand. J. Rehab. Med.* **13**: 12–20.

Halkjaer-Kristensen, J., and Ingemann-Hansen, T. (1985d) Wasting of the human quadriceps muscle after knee ligament injuries: III, oxidative and glycolytic enzyme activities. *Scand. J. Rehab. Med.* **13**: 21–28.

Harman, E. (1994) The biomechanics of resistance exercise. In *Essentials of Strength Training and Conditioning*, edited by T. R. Baechle, Human Kinetics: Champaign, IL, pp. 19–50.

Hather, B. M., Adams, G. R., Tesch, P. A., and Susley, G. A. (1992) Skeletal muscle responses to lower limb suspension in humans. *J. Appl. Physiol.* **72**: 1493–1498.

Henriksson, J., and Reitman, J. S. (1977) Time course of changes in human skeletal muscle succinate dehydrogenase and cytochrome oxidase activities and maximal oxygen uptake with physical activity and inactivity. *Acta Physiol. Scand.* **99**: 91–97.

Hislop, H. J. (1964) Response of immobilized muscle to isometric exercise. *J. Am. Phys. Ther. Assoc.* **44**: 339–347.

Houmard, J. A., Hortobagyi, T., Johns, R. A., Bruno, N. L., Nute, C.C., Shinebarger, M. H., and Welborn, J. W. (1992) Effect of short-term training cessation on performance measures in distance runners. *Int. J. Sports Med.* **13**: 572–576.

Houmard, J. A., Hortobagyi, T., Neufer, P. D., Johns, R. A., Fraser, D. D., Israel, R. G., and Dohm, G. L. (1993) Training cessation does not alter GLUT-4 protein levels in human skeletal muscle. *J. Appl. Physiol.* **74**: 776–781.

Houston, M. E., Bentzen, H., and Larsen, H. (1979) Interrelationships between skeletal muscle adaptations and performance as studied by detraining and retraining. *Acta Physiol. Scand.* **105**: 163–170.

Houston, M. E., Froese, E. A., Valeriote, S. P., Green, H. J., and Ranney, D. A. (1983) Muscle performance, morphology and metabolic capacity during strength training and detraining: a one leg model. *Eur. J. Appl. Physiol.* **51**: 25–35.

Ingemann-Hansen, T., and Halkjaer-Kristensen, J. (1977) Lean and fat component of the human thigh: the effects of immobilization in plaster and subsequent physical training. *Scand. J. Rehab. Med.* **9**: 67–72.

Ingemann-Hansen, T., and Halkjaer-Kristensen, J. (1980) Computerized tomographic determination of human thigh components. *Scand. J. Rehab. Med.* **12**: 27–31.

Jansson, E., Sylven, C., Arvidsson, I., and Eriksson, E. (1987) Increase in myoglobin content and decrease in oxidative enzyme activities by leg muscle immobilization in man. *Acta Physiol. Scand.* **132**: 515–517.

Jenkins, D. G., Imms, F. J., Prestidge, S. P., and Small, G. I. (1976) Muscle strength before and after meniscectomy: a comparison of methods of post-operative management. *Rheumatol. Rehab.* **15**: 153–155.

Kannus, P., Jozsa, L., Renstrom, P., Jarvinen, M., Kvist, M., Lehto, M., Oja, P., and Vuori, I. (1992) The effects of training, immobilization and remobilization on musculoskeletal tissue. *Scand. J. Med. Sci. Sports.* **2**: 100–118.

Klausen, K., Andersen, L. B., and Pelle, I. (1980) Adaptive changes in work capacity, skeletal muscle capillarization and enzyme levels during training and detraining. *Acta Physiol. Scand.* **113**: 9–16.

Larsson, L., and Ansved, T. (1985) Effects of long-term physical training and detraining on enzyme histochemical and functional skeletal muscle characteristics in man. *Muscle Nerve* **8**: 714–722.

Lindboe, C. F., and Platou, C. S. (1982) Disuse atrophy of human skeletal muscle: an enzyme histochemical study. *Acta Neuropath.* **56**: 241–244.

MacDougall, J. D., Elder, G. C. B., Sale, D. G., Moroz, J. R., and Sutton, J. R. (1980) Effects of strength training and immobilization on human muscle fibres. *Eur. J. Appl. Physiol.* **43**: 23–34.

MacDougall, J. D., Ward, G. R., Sale, D. G., and Sutton, J. R. (1977) Biochemical adaptation of human skeletal muscle to heavy resistance training and immobilization. *J. Appl. Physiol.* **43**: 700–703.

McCoy, M., Proietto, J., and Hargreaves, M. (1994) Effect of detraining on GLUT-4 protein in human skeletal muscle. *J. Appl. Physiol.* **77**: 1532–1536.

Miles, M. P., Clarkson, P. M., Bean, M., Ambach, K., Mulroy, J., and Vincent, K. (1994) Muscle function at the wrist following 9 d of immobilization and suspension. *Med. Sci. Sports Exerc.* **26**: 615–623.

Moore, R. L., Thacker, E. M., Kelley, G. A., Musch, T. I., Sinoway, L. I., Foster, V. L., and Dickinson, A. L. (1987) Effect of training/detraining on submaximal exercise responses in humans. *J. Appl. Physiol.* **63**: 1719–1724.

Morrissey, M. C., Brewster, C. E., Shields, C. L., and Brown, M. (1985) The effects of electrical stimulation on the quadriceps during postoperative knee immobilization. *Am. J. Sports Med.* **13**: 40–46.

Narici, M. V., Roi, G. S., Minetti, A. E., and Cerretelli, P. (1989) Changes in force, cross-sectional area and neural activation during strength training and detraining of the human quadriceps. *Eur. J. Appl. Physiol.* **59**: 310–319.

Neuffer, P. D., Costill, D. L., Fielding, R. A., Flyn, M. G., and Kirwan, J. P. (1987) Effect of reduced training on muscular strength and endurance in competitive swimmers. *Med. Sci. Sports Exerc.* **19**: 486–490.

Orlander, J., Kiessling, K.-H., Karlsson, J., and Ekblom, B. (1977) Low intensity training, inactivity and resumed training in sedentary men. *Acta Physiol. Scand.* **101**: 351–362.

Pickering, G., Fellmann, N., Morio, B., Ritz, P., Amonchot, A., Vermorel, M., and Coudert, J. (1997) Effects of endurance training on the cardiovascular system and water compartments in the elderly. *J. Appl. Physiol.* **83**: 1300–1306.

Ploutz-Snyder, L. L., Tesch, P. A., Crittenden, D. J., and Dudley, G. A. (1995) Effect of unweighting on skeletal muscle use during exercise. *J. Appl. Physiol.* **79**: 168–175.

Rennie, M. J., Edwards, R. H. T., Emery, P. W., Halliday, D., Lundholm, K., and Millward, D. J. (1983) Depressed protein synthesis is the dominant characteristic of muscle wasting and cachexia. *Clin. Physiol.* **3**: 387–398.

Richter, E. A., Kiens, B., Mizuno, M., and Strange, S. (1989) Insulin action in human thighs after one-legged immobilization. *J. Appl. Physiol.* **67**: 19–23.

Sale, D. G., McComas, J., MacDougall, J. D., and Upton, A. R. M. (1982) Neuromuscular adaptation in human thenar muscles following strength training and immobilization. *J. Appl. Physiol.* **53**: 419–424.

Sargeant, A. J., Davies, C. T. M., Edwards, R. H. T., Maunder, C., and Young, A. (1977) Functional and structural changes after disuse of human muscle. *Clin. Sci. Mol. Med.* **52**: 337–342.

Shaver, L. G. (1973) Cross transfer effects of training and detraining on relative muscle endurance. *Am. Corr. Ther. J.* **27**: 49–56.

Shaver, L. G. (1975) Cross training effects of conditioning and deconditioning on muscular strength. *Ergonomics* **18**: 9–16.

Simsolo, R. B., Ong, J. M., and Kern, P. A. (1993) The regulation of adipose tissue and muscle lipoprotein lipase in runners by detraining. *J. Clin. Invest.* **92**: 2124–2130.

Stillwell, D. M., McLarren, G. L., and Gersten, J. W. (1967) Atrophy of quadriceps muscle due to immobilization of the lower extremity. *Arch. Phys. Med. Rehab.* **48**: 289–295.

Sysler, B. L., and Stull, G. A. (1970) Muscular endurance retention as a function of length of detraining. *Res. Q. Exerc. Sport* **41**: 105–109.

Vaughan, V. G. (1989) Effects of upper limb immobilization on isometric muscle strength, movement time, and triphasic electromyographic characteristics. *Phys. Ther.* **69**: 119–129.

Vinnars, E., Bergstrom, J., Furst, P. (1975) Influence of the postoperative state on the intracellular free amino acids in human muscle tissue. *Ann. Surg.* **182**: 665–671.

Vukovich, M. D., Arciero, P. J., Kohrt, W. M., Racette S. B., Hansen, P. A., and Holloszy, J. O. (1996) Changes in insulin action and GLUT-4 with 6 days of inactivity in endurance runners. *J. Appl. Physiol.* **80**: 240–244.

Waldman, R., and Stull, G. A. (1969) Effects of various periods of inactivity on retention of newly acquired levels of muscular endurance. *Res. Q. Exerc. Sport* **40**: 396–401.

Ward, G. R., MacDougall, J. D., Sutton, J. R., Toews, C. J., and Jones, N. L. (1986) Activation of human muscle pyruvate dehydrogenase with activity and immobilization. *Clin. Sci.* **70**: 207–210.

White, M. J., and Davies, C. T. M. (1984) The effects of immobilization, after lower leg fracture, on the contractile properties of human triceps surae. *Clin. Sci.* **66**: 277–282.

White, M. J., Davies, C. T. M., and Brooksby, P. (1984) The effects of short-term voluntary immobilization on the contractile properties of the human triceps surae. *Q. J. Exp. Physiol.* **69**: 685–691.

Wolf, E., Magora, A., and Gonen, B. (1971) Disuse atrophy of the quadriceps muscle. *Electromyography* **11**: 479–490.

Wroblewski, R., Arvidsson, I., Eriksson, E., and Jansson, E. (1987) Changes in elemental composition of human muscle fibers following surgery and immobilization: an X-ray microanalytical study. *Acta Physiol. Scand.* **130**: 491–494.

Young, A., Hughes, I., Round, J. M., and Edwards, R. H. T. (1982) The effect of knee injury on the number of muscle fibers in the human quadriceps femoris. *Clin. Sci.* **62**: 227–234.

CHAPTER 5

Free Radical Processes in Conditioning and Deconditioning

Józef Kędziora

Department of Biochemistry, The Ludwik Rydygier Medical University, Bydgoszcz, Poland

> Unlearn'd he knew no schoolman's subtle art,
> No language, but language of the heart.
> By nature honest, by experience wise,
> Healthy by temp'rance, and by exercise.
>
> *Alexander Pope*

INTRODUCTION

The normal functioning of the body depends on many levels of homeostasis, one of which involves a balance between the generation of reactive oxygen species (ROS) and other free radicals and the anti-oxidant defense mechanisms (Table 5.1). This balance is, of course, dynamic and variable as the state of the body changes. One can ask at which point during normal physical activity is the equilibrium established; the obvious expectation would be that this point should usually correspond to the limited low level of physical activity that is necessary to perform the vital functions of an individual. Physical activity of high intensity means increases in metabolism which augments production of free radicals and other reactive oxygen species and increases oxidative stress. Interestingly, an opposite situation; that is, immobilization, is also outside the optimal physiological range of physical activity of an organism and can be expected to result in a dissociation between the formation and removal of reactive oxygen species. Contrary to intuitive expectations, however, studies of both extreme situations indicate that intensive physical activity and significant immobilization deconditioning (namely, bed rest) instigate oxidative stress. In this chapter I would like to discuss tentative explanations for these findings.

Table 5.1   Main reactive oxygen species formed in the body and main anti-oxidant mechanisms (free radicals in italics)

Reactive oxygen species (ROS)	Anti-oxidant defense means

Superoxide radical anion $O_2^{-\circ}$
Hydrogen peroxide H_2O_2
Hydroxyl radical $^\circ OH$
Singlet oxygen $^1O_2$
Peroxynitrite $ONOO^-$
Hypochlorite OCl^-
	Anti-oxidants:
	  Glutathione
	  Ascorbic acid (vitamin C)
	  Tocopherol (vitamin E)
	  Carotenoids

	Enzymes disposing of ROS:
	  Superoxide dismutase
	  Catalase
	  Glutathione peroxidase/glutathione reductase
	  Thioredoxin/thioredoxin reductase/thio-
	  redoxin peroxidase

PHYSICAL EXERCISE AND CONDITIONING

Whole-body physical exercise requires a considerable increase in metabolism, including the oxidative metabolism; intensity of whole-body respiration is augmented 10–15-fold (Keul et al., 1996). However, oxygen flux in the active peripheral skeletal muscle tissue may increase by about 100-fold with an approximate 30-fold increase in blood flow and about a threefold increase in arteriovenous-oxygen difference (Sen, 1995). Superoxide anions are released in the mitochondria as by-products of mitochondrial respiration. Up to 4% of the oxygen utilized by mitochondria is not reduced to water in a four-electron pathway, but only to superoxide via a one-electron pathway. Therefore, intensification of mitochondrial respiration means rapid augmentation of ROS production that is not compensated appropriately by anti-oxidant mechanisms. Because these anti-oxidant mechanisms are adapted metabolically to a more quiescent situation, oxidative stress intensifies. Oxidative stress has been measured in isolated pigeon heart mitochondria; the rate of superoxide anion production increases in direct proportion to the rate of mitochondrial oxygen consumption (Boveris and Chance, 1973). Another important source of ROS during exercise may be the oxidation of catecholamines and infiltration of muscles by neutrophils which release superoxide radical anions, hydrogen peroxide, nitrous oxide, and hypochlorite. Strenuous exercise causes an influx of neutrophils into muscle tissues (Belcastro et al., 1996; Ohishi et al., 1998). The pathophysiological mechanism of ischemia-reperfusion during strenous exercise, especially with accumulation of hypoxanthine and activation of xanthine oxidase, may also contribute to the tissue damage caused by ROS (Hellsten, 1993; Packer, 1997).

    Muscle tissue may be especially sensitive to oxidative damage because the anti-oxidant defenses of skeletal muscles and heart are poor. Basal metabolism of the heart is about 100% higher than that of the liver. At rest, a kilogram of human heart or liver tissue was estimated to consume oxygen at rates of 94 and 44 ml·min^{-1}, respectively (Diem and Lentner, 1970). In men, the activities of superoxide dismutase and catalase are, respectively, 16 and 40 times higher in the liver than in gastrocnemius muscle (Jenkins et al., 1984).

Exercise is accompanied by increased steady-state levels of tissue-free radicals and other reactive oxygen species. The content of free radicals in muscles, estimated by electron spin resonance (ESR) spectrometry, increased by 70% during exercise compared with their content at rest (Jackson et al., 1985). Other data confirmed that exhaustive treadmill exercise enhanced free radicals in muscle and liver by two- to threefold (Dillard et al., 1978; Davies et al., 1982). Exhaustive swimming exercise increased ESR signals of free radicals in rat myocardium (Kumar et al., 1992). These studies utilizing direct ESR spectroscopy were confirmed by employing the spin trapping attitude (Somani, 1994).

There is abundant evidence of oxidative stress during physical exercise. Whole-body exercise in both humans (Dillard et al., 1978; Balke et al., 1984; Maughan et al., 1989) and rats (Gee and Tappel, 1981; Goldfarb et al., 1994) results in augmented lipid peroxidation. Physical exercise in humans at 75% of the maximal oxygen uptake ($\dot{V}O_{2\,max}$) increased the level of expired pentane (a final product of lipid peroxidation) by 80% compared with that from resting subjects (Dillard et al., 1978). Lipid peroxidation also increased in humans performing submaximal (50% $\dot{V}O_{2\,max}$) exercise (Balke et al., 1984). The concentrations of expired pentane and serum malondialdehyde (MDA), which are end-products of lipid peroxidation, were elevated during submaximal (60% $\dot{V}O_{2\,max}$) exercise and increased further with increasing oxygen levels (Kanter et al., 1993). Hepatic lipid peroxidation increased by 220% in mouse liver (Leeuwenburgh and Ji, 1995). Concentrations of lipid peroxidation products in blood plasma increase during exercise (Kanter et al., 1993; Lovlin et al.,1987; Sen et al., 1994), although some authors found no appreciable changes (Kretzschmar et al., 1991). The highest lipid peroxidation was observed at maximal oxygen uptake (Viguie et al., 1990). Half-marathon exercise resulted in increased erythrocyte susceptibility to peroxidation (Duthie et al., 1990). Exercise at 50% and 77% $\dot{V}O_{2\,max}$ increased blood plasma lipid peroxidation products that were determined to be thiobarbituric acid-reactive substances (TBARS) (Sen et al., 1994).

Other indices of oxidative stress after intensive physical exercise include oxidation of DNA bases, decreased content of reduced glutathione (GSH), and an increase in the oxidized (GSSG) to reduced glutathione ratio (GSSG/GSH) (Packer, 1997). A sharp increase in blood and plasma GSSG was observed after human exercise (Gohil et al., 1988), and the total glutathione content in muscle decreased (Sen et al., 1993). An acute bout of prolonged exercise decreased liver GSH content by as much as 30% in rats (Lew et al., 1985) and mice (Leeuwenburgh and Ji, 1995). Myocardial GSH content was decreased by over 20% after mice swam to exhaustion (Leeuwenburgh et al., 1996). These findings reflect a change in the redox state of glutathione after exercise; on the other hand they suggest that oxidized glutathione can be actively pumped out of skeletal muscle and the heart during exercise (Sen, 1995; Ji and Leeuwenburgh, 1995). Such an active export of oxidized glutathione is a protective mechanism, for an accumulation of GSSG is harmful to the cell. Data on the behavior of blood GSH during exercise are contradictory. Some authors observed no change of blood GSH during intensive exercise (Garin, 1983; Ji et al., 1993), whereas others noted a sharp fall in blood GSH within the first 15 min of bicycling at 65% $\dot{V}O_{2\,max}$ (Gohil et al., 1988; Viguie et al., 1993). Half-marathon (Duthie et al., 1990) and 12-km running (Ohtsuka et al., 1994) decreased erythrocyte reduced-glutathione, and exercising at 50% and 77% $\dot{V}O_{2\,max}$ increased the blood GSSG/GSH ratio (Sen et al., 1994). Exhaustive exercise also decreased erythrocyte glutathione reductase in horses (Brady et al., 1977). No change in total plasma anti-oxidant capacity was observed during exercise (Sen et al., 1994) which may be the result of significant increases in blood plasma uric acid (Sjödin and Westing, 1990) and ascorbate (Viguie et al., 1993), two important contributors to the plasma anti-oxidant capacity.

Exercising at 50% and 77% $\dot{V}O_{2\,max}$ induces deoxyribonucleic acid (DNA) damage in blood leukocytes as assessed by fluorimetric analysis of DNA unwinding (Sen et al., 1994). In mammals, oxidative DNA damage appears to be correlated with metabolic rate (Ames et al., 1993); the increased exercise metabolism can be expected to augment the rate of damage. The level of oxidized DNA bases increased by 30% over the resting level 10 hr after marathon running (Aslan et al., 1997; Alessio, 1993).

Another target for oxidative stress is the proteins, especially the aromatic and sulfur amino acid residues. There is evidence for skeletal muscle protein oxidation in rats during exhaustive exercise (Reznick et al., 1992). Skeletal muscle microsomes contained fewer protein thiol groups and showed extensive protein cross-linking after exercise (Rajguru et al., 1994). Among the proteins that are targets for ROS are the anti-oxidant enzymes themselves, which are also inactivated by ROS (Blum and Fridovich, 1985; Pigeolet et al., 1990). Maximal exercise caused a decrease in glutathione peroxidase and catalase activities in the muscles of calcium-deficient rats, apparently a result of this mechanism (Oh-ishi et al., 1998). These data also point to the role of nutritional factors in determining the effects of physical exercise. Whole blood glutathione peroxidase was lowered in untrained subjects after acute exercise (Aslan et al., 1997) and erythrocyte catalase activity decreased after a 12-km run (Ohtsuka et al., 1994).

It has been suggested that oxidative stress contributes to oxidative skeletal muscle fatigue (Barclay and Hansel, 1991) and to muscular atrophy (Kondo and Itokawa, 1994). Xanthine oxidase may be the main source of superoxide radicals responsible for muscle fatigue; however, this mechanism seems to involve generation of the hydroxyl radical since the effect was attenuated by iron chelation or scavenging of the hydroxyl radical (Barclay and Hansel, 1991).

Physical exercise also releases iron; that is, increasing the pool of "loosely bound iron" (Jenkins et al., 1993; Jenkins, 1993) which may participate in the Fenton reaction (between hydrogen peroxide and Fe^{2+}) generating the most dangerous reactive oxygen species—the hydroxyl radical. The increased release of iron leads, in turn, to whole-body iron loss which may result in "sports anemia" (Ehn et al., 1980; Haymes, 1987).

The disturbance of the pro-oxidant/anti-oxidant balance by physical exercise, especially exertion that is long-lasting and repeated regularly (training), may induce an adaptive reaction bringing balance back to the equilibrium point by increasing anti-oxidants and anti-oxidant enzymes. Exercise training in rats increases activity of both Cu, Zn-superoxide dismutase (SOD) (Higuchi et al., 1985) and Mn-SOD in muscles and several other organs (Pereira et al., 1992). Rats trained to swim over a 10-week period increased the activities of glutathione peroxidase and glutathione reductase, as well as the overall anti-oxidant capacity of muscle, heart, and liver. The level of GSH can also be increased in rat muscle after training, whereas vitamin E level was unchanged in several tissues (Venditti and DiMeo, 1996). Such training also increased total anti-oxidant capacity in muscle, heart, and liver (Venditti and DiMeo, 1997). Long-term (18.5-month) endurance training of rats increased cardiac catalase and decreased the malondialdehyde (MDA) content of cardiac mitochondria (Kim et al., 1996). Interestingly, lipid peroxidation increased after 20 min of exercise in white muscle, but not in the red muscle of trained rats (Alessio and Goldfarb, 1989). In another study, 10 weeks of exercise training of rats did not increase anti-oxidative enzyme activities, but decreased the MDA level with respect to nontrained animals (Fiebig et al., 1996). Swim training (21 weeks) increased catalase activity in mouse heart (Kanter et al., 1985). Eight weeks of treadmill-running exercise training increased cytosolic and mitochondrial glutathione peroxidase activities in rat skeletal muscles (Ji, 1993). Sprint training of rats increased the total glutathione content of skeletal muscles and the activity of glutathione peroxidase in heart and skeletal muscles, but had no effect on superoxide activity in either heart or skeletal muscles (Sen, 1995). Modulation of anti-oxidant status is not confined to muscle. Nine-week training of rats resulted in augmented activity of catalase in muscles, testes, lung, liver, and brain (where the increase was highest—by 350%), and glutathione peroxidase in lungs, liver, and brain, and glutathione reductase in the testes. The adaptation was tissue-specific. Ten-week treadmill training of rats increased GSH content by 33%, the activity of glutathione peroxidase by 62%, and superoxide dismutase by 27% in deep vastus lateralis muscle; in soleus muscle the GSH level decreased and activities of glutathione peroxidase and superoxide dismutase remained unchanged (Leeuwenburgh et al., 1997). Exercise training also altered the kinetic properties of anti-oxidant enzymes (Somani and Husain, 1996); a result more difficult to interpret, and possibly a result of post-translational modifications.

Data on the adaptive increases in activities of SOD and glutathione peroxidase in rodent diaphragm and SOD in ventricular myocardium indicated that moderate-to-high intensity long-duration exercise is necessary to induce these changes (Powers et al., 1993; Powers and Criswell, 1996). These findings cause some doubt about any beneficial action of occasional physical activity ("weekend athletes") for increasing anti-oxidant potential of the body (Clarkson, 1995).

Increased concentrations of anti-oxidants and augmented anti-oxidant enzyme activities have also been reported in rats and trained humans (Jenkins et al., 1984; Caldarera et al., 1973; Tessier et al., 1995a,b; Mena et al., 1991; Duthie, 1996; Robertson et al., 1991; Ortenblad et al., 1997; Rokitzki et al., 1994). Exercise training increased catalase activity in rat liver, heart, and skeletal muscle (Caldarera et al., 1973). Comparison of trained, high-aerobic-capacity subjects ($\dot{V}O_{2\,max} > 60$

ml·kg^{-1}·min^{-1}) and low-fit subjects ($\dot{V}O_{2\,max}$ < 60 ml ·kg^{-1}·min^{-1}) showed that the high-fit group had significantly higher activities of superoxide dismutase and catalase activities in the vastus lateralis muscle (needle biopsy samples). Moreover, there was a positive correlation between the $\dot{V}O_{2\,max}$ and muscle catalase and super-oxide activities (r = 0.72 and 0.60, respectively, Jenkins et al., 1984). Ten-week endurance training increased plasma and erythrocyte glutathione peroxidase activities, but reduced erythrocyte glutathione reductase activity (Tessier et al., 1995a). Twenty-day intensive cycling (2,800 km) increased erythrocyte SOD activity (Mena et al., 1991), and an increase in erythrocyte glutathione content was observed in subjects who trained daily by running over a period of at least 2 years (Duthie, 1996). Exercise training of runners resulted in increases of erythrocyte α-tocopherol content and lymphocyte ascorbic acid concentrations. Erythrocyte glutathione peroxidase and catalase activities were positively correlated significantly with the weekly training distance (Robertson et al., 1991). Jump-trained humans also had higher levels of anti-oxidant enzymes (SOD, glutathione peroxidase, and glutathione reductase) in muscle (Ortenblad et al., 1997). Data from another study revealed negative correlations between individual aerobic capacity and resting plasma MDA level ($r = -0.82$), and exercise-induced increase in plasma MDA level ($r = -0.81$); these correlations suggest a beneficial effect of physical fitness (Sen, 1995). The serum level of TBARS decreased in trained athletes after extreme endurance stress (Rokitzki et al., 1994).

It has been hypothesized that the increased rate of free radical production or the release of some by-products of free radical formation are stimuli for induction of anti-oxidant enzymes (Ji et al., 1990). One can expect that the increase in activities of anti-oxidant enzymes and, indirectly, increases in the concentrations of anti-oxidants may be mediated by redox-regulated transcription factors such as NF-κB (Mihm et al., 1995). Our findings also point to another mechanism: increases in the activities of anti-oxidant enzymes (Cu, Zn-SOD, glutathione peroxidase, and catalase) and diminution of erythrocyte malondialdehyde (MDA) concentration in the erythrocytes of exercise-trained subjects during maximal exercise; no such increase was observed in subjects with low physical endurance (Blaszczyk et al., 1993, 1994a, 1994b; Sibińska et al., 1997). Similar changes were observed in blood platelets (Buczyński et al., 1990, 1991). After 40-min of exercise at 60% $\dot{V}O_{2\,max}$ in healthy individuals, glutathione peroxidase increased; in diabetics it decreased (Atalay et al., 1997). A postexercise increase in whole-blood glutathione peroxidase in exercise-trained subjects was found (Aslan et al., 1997). Treadmill exercise increased erythrocyte SOD, glutathione peroxidase, and catalase activities (Das et al., 1993), and cycling exercise at 70% $\dot{V}O_{2\,max}$ increased the blood glutathione reductase and glutathione released from the liver into the blood. Exercise with carbo-hydrate supplementation also increased blood glutathione peroxidase and glucose 6-phosphate dehydrogenase (Ji et al., 1993); also, muscle glutathione peroxidase increased after acute (submaximal + maximal) exercise in trained, but not in untrained, subjects (Tessier et al., 1995b). Glutathione reductase was increased by treadmill running (60% $\dot{V}O_{2\,max}$) in female athletes (Kanaley and Ji, 1991). In rats subjected to maximal exercise, erythrocyte catalase activity increased during swimming for up to 6 hr (Tanayeva et al., 1979). Erythrocyte anti-oxidant enzyme activities (SOD, catalase, and glutathione peroxidase) decreased after 60 min of cycling (70% $\dot{V}O_{2\,max}$) in an untrained group, but these decreases did not occur in endurance-trained subjects (Toskulkao and Glinsukon, 1996), a result partly compatible with our findings. These changes may be a result of altered intracellular milieu or of a release of younger blood cells from depots; nevertheless, they may represent an anti-oxidant mechanism mobilized during exercise.

Beneficial effects of activation of an anti-oxidant defense are not limited to physical exercise: they also include increased resistance of rats to ischemia and reperfusion injury (known to be dependent on anti-oxidant defense) after exercise training (Libonati et al., 1997; Bersohn and Scheuer, 1978; Kihlstrom, 1990); and physical activity in humans is associated with reduced morbidity and mortality from ischemic heart disease (Blair et al., 1989; Morris et al., 1980). These data support the positive health effects of physical exercise.

However, decreased generation of ROS by granulocytes occurs in exercise-trained subjects, and is inversely related to their level of physical conditioning (Nieman, 1994). The physiological sequelae of this inverse effect may be harmful as decreased ROS generation impairs the defensive capacity of phagocytes, and trained sportsmen appear to be more prone to upper respiratory tract infections (Peters, 1997).

Numerous though not unequivocal data indicate that anti-oxidant supplementation may reduce indices of oxidative stress after intense physical exercise (Jackson et al., 1985; Dillard et al., 1978; Davies et al., 1982; Warren et al., 1992). In exercising rats, vitamin E supplementation reduced the levels of lipid hydroperoxides and TBARS in blood plasma (Goldfarb et al., 1994; Reznick et al., 1992; Brady et al., 1979), liver, heart, blood, and skeletal muscle (Reznick et al., 1992). Similar results were obtained in humans (Sumida et al., 1989), including decreased pentane exhalation during high-altitude exposure in the Himalayas (Gerster, 1991). There is a protective effect of vitamin E on exercise-induced protein oxidation in skeletal muscle (Reznick et al., 1992), and urinary and muscle lipid peroxidation products were lower in vitamin E-supplemented subjects (Meydani et al., 1993). N-acetylcysteine (NAC) has anti-oxidant properties in that it scavenges free radicals and acts as a proglutathione drug, thereby providing cysteine for glutathione biosynthesis; apparently it has no side effects in humans (Arouma et al., 1989). Not surprisingly, NAC significantly decreased exercise-induced blood glutathione oxidation in humans and rats (Sen, 1995; Sen et al., 1994a,b). Vitamin C supplementation reduced the post-exercise decrease in muscle force observed in trained subjects (Jakeman and Maxwell, 1993). Administration of exogenous glutathione considerably increased (by 100–140%) the endurance of mice to physical exercise (Cazzulani et al., 1991; Novelli et al., 1991), and similar effects of vitamin E and spin-trapping agents were observed in these animals (Novelli et al., 1990).

Supplementation with anti-oxidant mixtures may be even more efficient. Results from human studies showed that administering a vitamin mixture containing β-carotene, vitamin C, and vitamin E for 5 weeks decreased lipid peroxidation both at rest and after physical exercise at 60% and 90% $\dot{V}O_{2\,max}$ (Kanter et al., 1993); and protected erythrocytes and skeletal muscle from exercise-induced injury (Witt et al., 1992). It did not, however, attenuate muscle damage in subjects exercising at 65% of maximal heart rate (Kanter and Eddy, 1992).

It has been reported that anti-oxidant supplementation not only attenuates the oxidative stress of physical exercise, but also improves the physical efficiency of exercising humans and animals. *In vitro* experimental data showed that the anti-oxidant N-acetylcysteine inhibited development of acute fatigue of rat diaphragm muscle fiber bundles (Khawli and Reid, 1994). Anti-oxidant vitamin supplementation can be recommended for individuals performing regular heavy exercise (Dekkers et al., 1996). On the other hand, anti-oxidant deficiency diminished and supplementation had beneficial effects on physical endurance; for example, vitamin E-deficient animals had reduced physical endurance (Davies et al., 1982; Packer, 1984; Goldfarb and Sen, 1994) and also showed increased lipid peroxidation, increased susceptibility of skeletal muscle to damage, and decreased oxidative phosphorylation in the liver (Goldfarb and Sen, 1994). Glutathione depletion compromised long-duration treadmill running performance (Sen, Atalay, and Hänninen, 1994) and swimming endurance in mice which suggests that glutathione homeostasis is essential for the pro-oxidant anti-oxidant balance during exercise (Sen, 1995). In humans, vitamin E supplementation for 1.5 months accelerated recovery from downhill-run-induced muscle damage (Cannon et al., 1990). Data on vitamin C are more contradictory: vitamin C supplementation did not alter run-time to exhaustion in vitamin E-deficient rats (Gohil et al., 1986), but 2 weeks of vitamin C supplementation attenuated the exercise-induced increase in lipid peroxidation in humans (Goldfarb and Sen, 1994).

In summary, the beneficial effects of activating the anti-oxidant defense by exercise conditioning are not limited to physical exercise: they may also include increased resistance to ischemia and reperfusion injury and to ischemic heart disease. Data support the positive health effects of physical exercise. Supplementation with anti-oxidants and anti-oxidant mixtures attenuates the free-radical injury induced by exercise and improves the physical efficiency of exercising persons. Anti-oxidant vitamin supplementation can be recommended for individuals performing regular heavy exercise.

IMMOBILIZATION AND BED REST DECONDITIONING

It seems surprising that severe limitation of physical exercise; namely, partial immobilization during prolonged bed rest (BR), also results in symptoms of oxidative stress. This problem may be pertinent to spaceflight deconditioning in relation to reduced physical exercise. In flight, moreover, astronauts are exposed to an increased flux of cosmic radiation, and there is 100% oxygen in the extravehicular mobility unit; both are sources of free radicals.

Men subjected to −4.5 degree head-down-tilt BR for 120 days showed increased lipid peroxidation in skeletal muscle, myocardium, and plasma which reached a peak at day 3 and remained elevated at day 60. Erythrocyte SOD decreased gradually during the 120-day BR period, whereas catalase activity showed some initial increase (day 28), then decreased significantly by day 72, and was normal at day 111 (Zezerov et al., 1989). Our studies on otherwise healthy persons who were immobilized with fractures of their lower extremities showed: decreased activity of Cu, Zn-SOD in erythrocytes on days 5, 12, 19, 26, and 40 of immobilization (maximally at day 12), decreased catalase activity during the entire immobilization period, decreased activity of glutathione peroxidase on day 5 and increased activity on day 19, and increased concentration of thiobarbituric acid-reactive substances (TBARS) after 5, 12, 19, 26, and 40 days of immobilization (Pawlak, 1998). Blood platelet activity of Cu, Zn-SOD, glutathione peroxidase and catalase were significantly decreased, and lipid peroxidation increased after 14 and 28 days of immobilization; later there was a tendency for normalization of all parameters studied after 90 days (Kędziora and Buczyński, 1996; Kafar et al., 1991a, b). One consequence of prolonged BR is decreased phagocytosis between days 8 and 14 (Greenleaf and Kozlowski, 1982). Because activated phagocytes are an important source of ROS, this decreased effect also contributed to diminished ROS generation during BR. We observed, in BR subjects, decreased basal superoxide generation by circulating granulocytes after 5, 12, 19, and 26 days, decreased superoxide generation after zymosan stimulation on days 12, 19, and 26; and decreased nitric oxide release from granulocytes (both basal and after stimulation with opsonized zymosan)—the decrease being maximal on day 12 (Pawlak, 1998).

Similar results were obtained in animals. Immobilization decreased catalase activity in rat erythrocytes (Taneyeva et al., 1979); and rats immobilized in a tilted −15 degree head-down position showed increased content of lipid peroxidation products, most notably in blood serum and skeletal muscles. After 60 days of immobilization the content of lipid peroxidation products in plasma decreased, but was still higher than that in the control group; it remained high in the liver. Shidlovskaya (1985) also showed a progressive increase in lipid peroxidation in skeletal muscle and heart of rats throughout immobilization. The intensity of this process increased with time of immobilization. After a 7-day flight in the Kosmos 1667 spaceship, rats showed no changes in plasma MDA concentrations or increased anti-oxidant capacity (Popova et al., 1988); but they had increased activity of total SOD (Cu, Zn-SOD plus Mn-SOD) in the heart and liver homogenates, unchanged SOD activity in muscle homogenates, decreased activity of glutathione peroxidase in skeletal muscles and liver (unchanged in the heart), and no changes of glutathione reductase or catalase activities; tocopherol concentration was higher in the heart and liver and lower in skeletal muscles, and MDA concentration was higher (by about 25%) in the liver and skeletal muscles and unchanged in the heart (Delenyan and Markin, 1989). However, it is probable that the increased gravitational stress during reentry from space could have affected these results. After a 13-day flight in the Kosmos 1887 spacecraft (Markin and Delenyan, 1992) and a 14-day flight in the Space 2044 spacecraft (Markin and Zhuhavleva, 1993), there was increased plasma malondialdehyde concentration and increased hepatic anti-oxidant enzyme activities in rats. In contrast, after an 8-day spaceflight (NASA Immune II Mission), rats showed decreased mRNA levels for Cu, Zn-SOD and glutathione peroxidase but unchanged activities of these enzymes; decreases in both mRNA levels and activities of catalase and glutathione reductase; considerable decreases in reduced, oxidized, and total glutathione concentration; and increased MDA content in the liver (Hollander and Gore, 1998). These results suggested that GSH could be considered as a dietary supplement during spaceflight. Cosmonauts who spent 4 to 13 days in space had decreased concentrations of vitamin E in their blood (Belakovsky et al., 1984). Immobilized rats showed decreased activity of cytochrome oxidase in the liver, skeletal muscles, kidneys, and brain on day 15 (Smirnov and Potapov, 1981); after 30 days there was a transient increase of cytochrome oxidase activity followed by a progressive decrease to day 60, and normalization on day 90. Cytochrome oxidase activity in the lungs was lower on day 60 and increased on day 90 (Smirnov and Potapov, 1981). Similar results on cytochrome oxidase were obtained in rats after spaceflight (Connor and Hood, 1998). Other authors have reported decreased activities of citric acid cycle enzymes in skeletal muscle (Potapov, 1989) and in liver (Ganin, 1983) of immobilized rats.

Interestingly, the pool of loosely bound iron was increased after immobilization of rat ankle in planar flexion for 4, 8, or 12 days. There was a significant increase in the soleus iron content and augmentation of TBARS and oxidized glutathione (GSSG) (Kondo et al., 1992a). The latter changes were suppressed by the iron chelator—deferoxamine (Kondo et al., 1992b).

Various mechanisms for the increased lipid peroxidation during deconditioning hypokinesia have been suggested including: increased activity of the hormonal component of the sympathicoadrenal system; accumulation of excessive quantities of free fatty acids; reduced activity of anti-oxidant enzymes; and increase in the amount of liberated adrenalin, autoxidation of which may be a source of ROS.

In brief we can conclude that: increased free-radical damage occurs during deconditioning hypokinesia; cosmonauts who spent several days in space had decreased levels of vitamin E in their blood; and anti-oxidants, among them gluta-thione, may be considered as dietary supplements during spaceflight.

SUMMARY AND POSSIBLE MECHANISMS

It is clear that both strenuous physical exercise and deconditioning–immobilization impose oxidative stress on the body, and that systematic exercise training augments anti-oxidative defense mechanisms in various tissues. In general, it seems that the occurrence of oxidative stress after immobilization is followed by apparent normali-zation of the parameters. These responses can be generalized in terms of pro-oxidant/ anti-oxidant homeostasis (Lewin and Popov, 1994) (homeoredox equilibrium, Figure 5.1). It assumes that in tissues and in the body there is a special level of homeostasis; that is, an equilibrium between pro-oxidative reactions and anti-oxidative defense reactions that prevents uncontrolled oxidative reactions. During exercise this balance is shifted toward oxidative stress that results in a compensatory

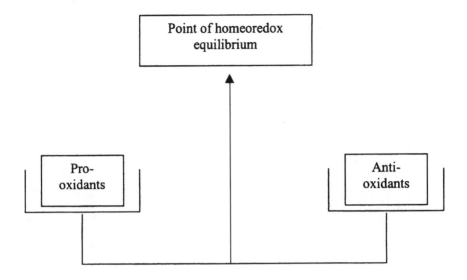

Figure 5.1 The idea of homeoredox equilibrium.

homeostatic response resulting in reestablishment of equilibrium at the expense of increased production of anti-oxidants and anti-oxidant enzymes. Means of attaining equilibrium may also include decreased production of ROS by phagocytes, an effect observed after exercise training.

During the first phase of immobilization the pro-oxidant anti-oxidant equilibrium is shifted toward a decrease in pro-oxidant reactions as a result of decreased oxygen consumption in the muscles. The homeoredox equilibrium is then reestablished by decreased concentration of anti-oxidants and decreased activities of anti-oxidant enzymes. If this process overshoots, a transient oxidative stress appears which, in turn, induces a compensatory increase of the anti-oxidant defenses that is observed after longer periods of immobilization.

PRACTICAL APPLICATIONS

One application of these findings would be prevention of oxidative damage during acute exercise. However, systemic administration of anti-oxidants during controlled exercise training seems less desirable; instead, the aim of systematic exercise training would be to increase the natural defense mechanisms of the body. Also, anti-oxidant supplementation would diminish the challenge of physical exercise in this respect. On the other hand, transient anti-oxidant supplementation might be appropriate during mobilization after BR deconditioning when the body is tuned to a lower level of pro-oxidant reaction and anti-oxidant defense and would adapt to an increased oxidative load.

Our health and longevity are conditioned by the robust but delicate balance between the pro-oxidant and anti-oxidant activities of the body. Regular physical exercise is beneficial in this respect in that it forces adaptation to physiological oxidative stress. This adaptation may prove useful in situations in which oxidative stress is caused by pathologic factors such as inflammation or ischemia-reperfusion. Since the system of pro-oxidant/anti-oxidant response is always tending toward a dynamic equilibrium, it should not be expected that increased anti-oxidant defense induced by exercise training will have a lasting effect; instead, its maintenance requires continuous systematic physical exercise.

REFERENCES

Alessio, H. M. (1993) Exercise-induced oxidative stress. *Med. Sci. Sports Exerc.* **25**: 218–224.

Alessio, H. M., and Goldfarb, A. H. (1989) Lipid peroxidation and scavenger enzymes during exercise: Adaptive response to training. *J. Appl. Physiol.* **64**: 1333–1336.

Ames, B. N., Shigenaga, M. K., and Hagen, T. M. (1993) Oxidants, antioxidants, and the degenerative diseases of aging. *Proc. Natl. Acad. Sci. USA* **90**: 7915–7922.

Aruoma, O. I., Halliwel, B., Hoey, B. M., and Butler, J. (1989) The antioxidant action of N-acetylcysteine: its reaction with hydrogen peroxide, hydroxyl radical, superoxide, and hypochlorous acid. *Free Radic. Biol. Med.* **6**: 593–597.

Aslan, R., Sekeroglu, M. R., Gultekin, F., and Bayiroglu, F. (1997) Blood lipoperoxidation and antioxidant enzymes in healthy individuals: relation to age, sex, habits, life style, and environment. *J. Environ. Sci. Health* **104A**: 2101–2109.

Atalay, M., Laaksonen, D. E., Niskanen, L., Uusitupa, M., Hänninen, O., and Sen, C. K. (1997) Altered antioxidant enzyme defences in insulin-dependent diabetic men with increased resting and exercise-induced oxidative stress. *Acta Physiol. Scand.* **161**: 195–201.

Balke, P. O., Snider, M. T., and Bull, A. P. (1984) Evidence for lipid peroxidation during moderate exercise. *Med. Sci. Sports Exerc.* **16**: 181 (Abstract).

Barclay, J. K., and Hansel, M. (1991) Free radicals may contribute to oxidative skeletal muscle fatigue. *Can. J. Physiol. Pharmacol.* **69**: 279–284.

Belakovsky, M. S., Radchenko, N. D., and Bogdanov, N. G. (1984) Vitamin metabolism in cosmonauts after short-term flights. *Kosm. Biol. Aviakosm. Med.* **18**: 19–22.

Belcastro, A. N., Arthur, G. D., Albisser, T. A., and Raj, D. A. (1996) Heart, liver, and skeletal muscle myeloperoxidase activity during exercise. *J. Appl. Physiol.* **80**: 1331–1335.

Bersohn, M. M., and Scheuer, J. (1978) Effect of ischemia on the performance of hearts from physically trained rats. *Am. J. Physiol.* **234**: 215–218.

Blair, S. N., Koho, H. W., Paffenbarger, R. S., Clark, D. G., Cooper, K. H., and Gibbons, L. W. (1989) Physical fitness and all-cause mortality: a prospective study of healthy men and women. *J.A.M.A.* **262**: 2395–2401.

Blaszczyk, J., Kędziora, H., Pastuszka, M., Sibińska, E., Kędziora, J., and Paśnik, J. (1994a) Wplyw submaksymalnego wysilku fizycznego na peroksydację lipidów oraz enzymatyczny uklad antyoksydacyjny w krwinkach czerwonych u ludzi zdrowych. *Wych. Fiz. Sport.* **1**: 53–60.

Blaszczyk, J., Sibińska, E., Kędziora, J., Kędziora-Kornatowska, K., Węclewska, U., and Paszkowski, J. (1993) Stopień peroksydacji lipidów oraz aktywność katalazy w krwinkach czerwonych u ludzi zdrowych podczas submaksymalnego wysilku fizycznego i restytucji. *Wych. Fiz. Sport.* **41**: 41–46.

Blaszczyk, J., Sibińska, E., Kędziora, J. et al. (1994b) Aktywność antyoksydacyjna i procesy peroksydacji lipidów w krwinkach czerwonych podczas submaksymalnego wysilku fizycznego. *Med. Sport.* **32**: 3–5.

Blum, J., and Fridovich, I. (1985) Inactivation of glutathione peroxidase by superoxide radical. *Arch. Biochem. Biophys.* **240**: 500–508.

Boveris, A., and Chance, B. (1973) The mitochondrial generation of hydrogen peroxide: general properties and effects of hyperbaric oxygen. *Biochem. J.* **134**: 707–716.

Brady, P. S., Brady, L. J., and Ulrey, D. E. (1979) Selenium, vitamin E, and the response to swimming stress in the rat. *J. Nutr.* **109**: 1103–1109.

Brady, P. S., Shelle, J. E., and Ullrey, D. E. (1977) Rapid changes in equine erythrocyte glutathione reductase with exercise. *Am. J. Vet. Res.* **38**: 1045–1048.

Buczyński, A., Kędziora, J., Blaszczyk, J., Kafar, K., Żolyński, K., and Nawarycz, T. (1990) Peroksydacja lipidów krwinek plytkowych u ludzi w stanie hipokinezji i po obciążeniu submaksymalnym wysilkiem fizycznym. *Wych. Fiz. Sport.* **34**: 43–49.

Buczyński, A., Kędziora, J., Tkaczewski, W., and Wachowicz, B. (1991) Effect of submaximal physical exercise on antioxidative protection of human blood platelets. *Int. J. Sports Med.* **12**: 52–54.

Caldarera, C. M., Guarnieri, C., and Lazzari, F. (1973) Catalase and peroxidase activity of cardiac muscle. *Boll. Soc. Ital. Biol. Sper.* **49**: 72–77.

Cannon, J. G., Orencole, S. F., Fielding, R. A. et al. (1990) Acute phase response in exercise: Interaction of age and vitamin E on neutrophils and muscle enzyme release. *Am. J. Physiol. Regulatory Integrative Comp. Physiol.* **259**: R1214–R1219.

Cazzulani, P., Cassin, M., and Ceserani, R. (1991) Increased endurance to physical exercise in mice given oral reduced glutathione (GSH). *Med. Sci. Res.* **19**: 543–544.

Clarkson, P. M. (1995) Antioxidants and physical performance. *Crit. Rev. Food Sci. Nutr.* **35**: 131–141.

Connor, M. K., and Hood, D. A. (1998) Effect of microgravity on the expression of mitochondrial enzymes in rat cardiac and skeletal muscles. *J. Appl. Physiol.* **84**: 593–598.

Das, S. K., Hinds, J. E., Hardy, R. E., Collins, J. C., and Mukherjee, S. (1993) Effects of physical stress on peroxide scavengers in normal and sickle cell trait erythrocytes. *Free Radic. Biol. Med.* **14**: 139–147.

Davies, K. J. A., Quintanilha, A. T., Brooks, G. A., and Packer, L. (1982) Free radicals and tissue damage produced by exercise. *Biochem. Biophys. Res. Comm.* **107**: 1198–1205.

Dekkers, J. C., Doornen, L. J., Kemper, H. C. (1996) The role of antioxidant vitamins and enzymes in the prevention of exercise-induced muscle damage. *Sports Med.* **21**: 213–238.

Delenyan, N. V., and Markin, A. A. (1989) Lipid peroxidation in rats after 7-day flight on Cosmos-1967. *Kosm. Biol. Aviakosm. Med.* **23**: 34–37.

Diem, K., and Lentner, C., editors (1970) *Scientific Tables. Documenta Geigy,* 7th ed., Geigy: Basel.

Dillard, C. J., Litov, R. E., Savin, W. M., and Tappel, A. L. (1978) Effects of exercise, vitamin E and ozone on pulmonary function and lipid peroxidation. *J. Appl. Physiol.* **45**: 927–932.

Duthie, G. G. (1996) Adaptations of the antioxidative defence system to chronic exercises. *Med. Sports Sci.* **41**: 95–101.

Duthie, G. G., Robertson, J. D., Maughan, R. J., and Morrice, P. C. (1990) Blood antioxidant status and erythrocyte lipid peroxidation following distance running. *Arch. Biochem. Biophys.* **282**: 78–83.

Ehn, L., Carlmark, B., and Hoglund, S. (1980) Ion status in athletes involved in intense physical activity. *Med. Sci. Sports Exerc.* **12**: 61–64.

Fiebig, R., Gore, M. T., Chandwaney, R., Leeuwenburgh, C., and Ji, L. L. (1996) Alteration of myocardial antioxidant enzyme activity and glutathione content with aging and exercise training. *Free Radic. Biol. Med.* **19**: 83–89.

Ganin, Y. A. (1983) Activity of oxidative enzymes of the tricarboxylic acid cycle in the liver of hypokinetic rats. *Kosm. Biol. Aviakosm. Med.* **17**: 67–71.

Gee, D. L., and Tappel, A. L. (1981) The effect of exhaustive exercise on expired pentane as a measure of in vivo lipid peroxidation in the rat. *Life Sci.* **28**: 2425–2429.

Gerster, H. (1991) Function of vitamin E in physical exercise: a review. *Z. Ernahrungswiss.* **30**: 89–97.

Gohil, K., Packer, L., De Lumen, B., Brooks, G. A., and Terblanche, S. E. (1986) Vitamin E deficiency and vitamin C supplements: exercise and mitochondrial oxidation. *J. Appl. Physiol.* **60**: 1986–1991.

Gohil, K., Viguie, C., Stanley, W. C., Brooks, G. A., and Packer, L. (1988) Blood glutathione oxidation during human exercise. *J. Appl. Physiol.* **64**: 115–119.

Goldfarb, A. H., McInstosh, M. K., Boyer, B. T., and Fatouros, J. (1994) Vitamin E effects on indexes of lipid peroxidation in muscle from DHEA-treated and exercised rats. *J. Appl. Physiol.* **76**: 1630–1635.

Goldfarb, A., and Sen, C. K. (1994) Antioxidant supplementation and the control of oxygen toxicity during exercise. In *Exercise and Oxygen Toxicity*, edited by C. K. Sen, L. Packer, and O. Hänninen, Elsevier: Amsterdam, pp.163–189.

Greenleaf, J. E., and Kozlowski, S. (1982) Physiological consequences of reduced physical activity during bed rest. *Exerc. Sport Sci. Rev.* **10**: 84–120.

Haymes, E. M. (1987) Nutritional concerns: need for iron. *Med. Sci. Sports Exerc.* **19**: 197–200.

Hellsten, Y. (1993) The role of xanthine oxidase in exercise. In *Exercise and Oxygen Toxicity,* edited by C. K. Sen, L. Packer, and O. Hänninen, Elsevier: Amsterdam, pp. 211–234.

Higuchi, M., Cartier, L. J., Chen, M., and Holoszy, J. O. (1985) Superoxide dismutase and catalase in skeletal muscle: adaptive response to exercise. *J. Gerontol.* **40**: 281–286.

Hollander, J., Gore, M. (1998) Spaceflight downregulates antioxidant defense systems in rat liver. *Free Radic. Biol. Med.* **24**: 385–390.

Jackson, M. J., Edwards, R. H. T., and Symons, M. R. C. (1985) Electron spin resonance studies of intact mammalian skeletal muscle. *Biochim. Biophys. Acta* **847**: 185–190.

Jakeman, P., and Maxwell, S. (1993) Effect of antioxidant vitamin supplementation on muscle function after eccentric exercise. *Eur. J. Appl. Physiol.* **67**: 426–430.

Jenkins, R. R. (1993) Exercise, oxidative stress, and antioxidants: a review. *Int. J. Sport Nutr.* **3**: 356–375.

Jenkins, R. R., Friedland, R., and Howald, H. (1984) The relationship of oxygen uptake to superoxide dismutase and catalase activity in human skletal muscle. *Int. J. Sports Med.* **5**: 11–14.

Jenkins, R. R., Krause, K., and Schofield, L. S. (1993) Influence of exercise on clearance of oxidant stress products and loosely bound iron. *Med. Sci. Sports Exerc.* **25**: 213–217.

Ji, L. L. (1993) Antioxidant enzyme response to exercise and aging. *Med. Sci. Sports Exerc.* **25**: 225–231.

Ji, L. L., Dillon, D., and Wu, E. (1990) Alteration of antioxidant enzymes with aging in rat skeletal muscle and liver. *Am. J. Physiol. Regulatory Integrative Comp. Physiol.* **258**: R918–R923.

Ji, L. L., Katz, A., Fu, R., Griffiths, M., and Spencer, M. (1993) Blood glutathione status during exercise: effect of carbohydrate supplementation. *J. Appl. Physiol.* **74**: 788–792.

Ji, L. L., and Leeuwenburgh, C. (1995) Exercise and glutathione. *In Pharmacology in Exercise and Sports*, edited by S. Somani, CRC: Boca Raton, FL, pp. 94–123.

Kafar, K., Buczyński, A., Żolyński, K., and Kędziora, J. (1991a) Stężenie dialdehydu malonowego (MDA) oraz aktywność dysmutazy ponadtlenkowej (SOD-1) w krwinkach plytkowych u osób w stanie dlugotrwalej hipokinezji. *Kwart. Ortoped.* **1**: 32–34, .

Kafar, K., Buczyński, A., Żolyński, K., and Kędziora, J. (1991b) Aktywność peroksydazy glutationowej (GPx) oraz katalazy (CAt) w krwinkach plytkowych u osób przebywających w stanie 28-dniowej hipokinezji. *Kwart. Ortoped.* **1**: 35–37.

Kanaley, J. A., and Ji, L. L. (1991) Antioxidant enzyme activity during prolonged exercise in amenorrheic and eumenorrheic athletes. *Metabolism* **40**: 88–92.

Kanter, M. M., and Eddy, D. D. (1992) Effect of antioxidant supplementation on serum markers of lipid peroxidation and skeletal muscle damage following eccentric exercise. *Med. Sci. Sports Exerc.* **24**: S17.

Kanter, M. M., Hamlin, R. R., Unverferth, D. V., Davis, M. V., and Merola, A. J. (1985) Effect of exercise training on antioxidant enzymes and cardiotoxicity of doxorubicin. *J. Appl. Physiol.* **59**: 1298–1303.

Kanter, M. M., Nolte, L. A., and Holloszy, J. O. (1993) Effects of an antioxidant vitamin mixture on lipid peroxidation at rest and post-exercise. *J. Appl. Physiol.* **74**: 965–969.

Kędziora, J., and Buczyński, A. (1996) Antioxidative enzyme activities and lipid peroxidation indicators in blood platelets during bed rest. *Int. J. Occup. Med. Environ. Health* **9**: 45–51.

Keul, J., Koenig, D., Huonker, M., and Berg, A. (1996) Nutrition, sport, and muscular stress tolerance. *Dtsch. Zeit. Sportmed.* **228**: 230–237.

Khawli, F. A., and Reid, M. B. (1994) N-Acetylcysteine depresses contractile function and inhibits fatigue of diaphragm in vitro. *J. Appl. Physiol.* **77**: 317–324.

Kihlstrom, M. (1990) Protection effect of endurance training against reoxygenation-induced injuries in rat heart. *J. Appl. Physiol.* **68**: 1672–1678.

Kim, J. D., Yu, B. P., McCarter, R. J., Lee, S. Y., and Herlihy, J. T. (1996) Exercise and diet modulate cardiac lipid peroxidation and antioxidant defenses. *Free Radic. Biol. Med.* **20**: 83–88.

Kondo, H., and Itokawa, Y. (1994) Oxidative stress in muscular atrophy. In *Exercise and Oxygen Toxicity*, edited by C. K. Sen, L. Packer, O. Hänninen, Elsevier: Amsterdam, pp. 319–342.

Kondo, H., Miura, M., Kodama, J., Ahmed, S. M., and Itokawa, Y. (1992a) Role of iron in oxidative stress in skeletal muscle atrophied by immobilization. *Pflügers Arch.* **421**: 295–297.

Kondo, H., Miura, M., Nakagaki, I., Sasaki, S., and Itokawa, Y. (1992b) Trace element movement and oxidative stress in skeletal muscle atrophied by immobilization. *Am. J. Physiol. Endocrinol. Metab.* **262**: E583–E590.

Kretzschmar, M., Müller, D., Hübscher, J., Marin, E., and Klinger, W. (1991) Influence of aging, training and acute exercise on plasma glutathione and lipid peroxides in man. *Int. J. Sports Med.* **12**: 218–222.

Kumar, C. T., Reddy, V. K., Prasad, M., Thyagaraju, K., and Reddanna, P. (1992) Dietary supplementation of vitamin E protects heart tissue from exercise-induced oxidant stress. *Mol. Cell. Biochem.* **111**: 109–115.

Leeuwenburgh, C., Hollander, J., Leichtweis, S., Griffiths, M., Gore, M., and Ji, L. L. (1997) Adaptations of glutathione antioxidant system to endurance training are tissue and muscle fiber specific. *Am. J. Physiol. Regulatory Integrative Comp. Physiol.* **272**: R363–R369.

Leeuwenburgh, C., and Ji, L. L. (1995) Glutathione depletion in rested and exercised mice: biochemical consequence and adaptation. *Arch. Biochem. Biophys.* **316**: 941–949.

Leeuwenburgh, C., Leichtweis, S., Hollander, J. R. F., Gore, M., and Ji, L. L. (1996) Effect of exercise on glutathione deficient heart. *Mol. Cell. Biochem.* **156**: 17–24.

Lew, H., Pyke, S., and Quintanilha, A. (1985) Changes in glutathione status of plasma, liver and muscle following exhaustive exercise in rats. *FEBS Lett.***185**: 262–266.

Lewin, G., and Popov, I. (1994) The antioxidant system of the organism. Theoretical basis and practical consequences. *Med. Hypoth.* **42**: 269–275.

Libonati, J. R., Gaughan, J. P., Hefner, C. A., Gow, A., Paolone, A. M., and Houser, S. R. (1997) Reduced ischemia and reperfusion injury following exercise training. *Med. Sci. Sports Exerc.* **29**: 509–516.

Lovlin, R., Cottle, W., Cavanagh, M., and Belcastro, A. L. (1987) Are indices of free radical damage related to exercise intensity? *Eur. J. Appl. Physiol.* **56**: 313–316.

Markin, A. A., and Delenyan, N. V. (1992) Lipid peroxidation and the system of antioxidant protection in rats following a 13-day spaceflight on the KOSMOS 1887 biosatellite. *Aviakosm. Ekologich. Med.* **26**: 43–50.

Markin, A. A., and Zhuhavleva, A. O. (1993) Lipid peroxidation and antioxidant defense system in rats after a 14-day spaceflight in the Space 2044 spacecraft. *Aviakosm. Ekologich. Med.* **27**: 47–50.

Maughan, R. J., Donnelly, A. E., Gleeson, M., Whiting, P. H., Walker, K. A., and Clough, P. J. (1989) Delayed-onset muscle damage and lipid peroxidation in man after a downhill run. *Muscle Nerve* **12**: 332–336.

Mena, P., Maynar, M., Gutierez, J. M., Maynar, J., Timon, J., and Campillo, J. E. (1991) Erythrocyte free radical scavenger enzymes in bicycle professional racers: adaptation to training. *Int. J. Sports Med.* **12**: 563–566.

Meydani, M., Evans, W. J., Handelman, G. et al. (1993) Protective effect of vitamin E on exercise-induced oxidative damage in young and older adults. *Am. J. Physiol. Regulatory Integrative Comp. Physiol.* **264**: R992–R998.

Mihm, S., Galter, D., and Droge, W. (1995) Modulation of transcription factor NF-kB activity by intracellular glutathione levels and by variations of extracellular cysteine supply. *FASEB J.* **9**: 246–252.

Morris, J. N., Pollard, R., Everitt, M. G., and Chave, S. P. W. (1980) Vigorous exercise in leisure-time: Protection against coronary heart disease. *Lancet* **2**: 1207–1210.

Nieman, D. (1994) Exercise, upper respiratory infections and the immune system. *Med. Sci. Sports Exerc.* **26**: 128–139.

Novelli, G. P., Bracciotti, G., and Falsini, S. (1990) Spin-trappers and vitamin E prolong endurance to muscle fatigue in mice. *Free Radic. Biol. Med.* **8**: 9–13.

Novelli, G. P., Falsini, S., and Bracciotti, G. (1991) Exogenous glutathione increases endurance to muscle effort in mice. *Pharmacol. Res.* **23**: 149–155.

Oh-ishi, S., Kizaki, T., Ookawara, T. et al. (1998) The effect of exhaustive exercise on the antioxidant enzyme system in skeletal muscle from calcium-deficient rats. *Pflügers Arch.* **435**: 767–774.

Ohtsuka, Y., Yabunaka, N., Fujisawa, H., Kamimura, H., and Agishi, Y. (1994) Effect of long-distance running and exercise with a bicycle ergometer on the erythrocyte antioxidative defense system. *Jpn. J. Phys. Fitness Sports Med.* **43**: 277–282.

Ortenblad, N., Madsen, K., and Djurhuus, M. S. (1997) Antioxidant status and lipid peroxidation after short-term maximal exercise in trained and untrained humans. *Am. J. Physiol. Regulatory Integrative Comp. Physiol.* **272**: R1258–R1263.

Packer, L. (1984) Vitamin E, physical exercise, and tissue damage in animals. *Med. Biol.* **62**: 105–109.

Packer, L. (1997) Oxidants, antioxidant nutrients and the athlete. *J. Sports Sci.* **15**: 353–363.

Pawlak, W. (1998) Effect of posttraumatic hypokinesia on the free radical processes and enzymatic antioxidant defense mechanisms. Doctoral Dissertation, *Military Medical University*, Łódź, Poland.

Pereira, B., Curi, R., Kokubun, E., and Bechara, E. J. H. (1992) 5-Aminolevulinic acid-induced alterations of oxidative metabolism in sedentary and exercise-trained rats. *J. Appl. Physiol.* **72**: 226–230.

Peters, E. M. (1997) Exercise, immunology, and upper respiratory tract infections. *Int. J. Sports Med.* **18** (Suppl. 1): S69–S77.

Pigeolet, E., Corbisier, P., Houbion, A. et al. (1990) Glutathione peroxidase, superoxide dismutase, and catalase inactivation by peroxides and oxygen-derived free radicals. *Mech. Ageing Dev.* **51**: 283–297.

Popova, I. A., Afonin, B. V., Vetrova, E. G. et al. (1988) Homeostatic reactions in blood of Cosmos-1667 rats. *Kosm. Biol. Aviakosm. Med.* **22**: 39–42.

Potapov, P. P. (1989) Changes in mitochondrial oxidative enzymes in rat skeletal muscles during recovery after hypokinesia of varying duration. *Kosm. Biol. Aviakosm. Med.* **23**:

65–67.

Powers, S. K., and Criswell, D. (1996) Adaptive strategies of respiratory muscles in response to endurance exercise. *Med. Sci. Sports Exerc.* **28**: 1115–1122.

Powers, S. K., Criswell, D., Lawler, J. et al. (1993) Rigorous exercise training increases superoxide dismutase activity in ventricular myocardium. *Am. J. Physiol. Heart Circ. Physiol.* **265**: H2094–H2098.

Rajguru, S. U., Yeargans, G. S., and Seidler, N. W. (1994) Exercise causes oxidative damage to rat skeletal muscle microsomes while increasing cellular sulfhydryls. *Life Sci.* **54**: 149–157.

Reznick, A. Z., Witt, E., Matsumoto, M., and Packer, L. (1992) Vitamin E inhibits protein oxidation in skeletal muscle of resting and exercise rats. *Biochem. Biophys. Res. Comm.* **189**: 801–806.

Robertson, J. D., Maughan, R. J., Duthie, G. G., and Morrice, P. C. (1991) Increased blood oxidant systems of runners in response to training load. *Clin. Sci.* **80**: 611–618.

Rokitzki, L., Logemann, E., Sagredos, A. N., Murphy, M., Wetzel-Roth, W., and Keul, J. (1994) Lipid peroxidation and antioxidative vitamins under extreme endurance stress. *Acta Physiol. Scand.* **151**: 149–158.

Sen, C. K. (1995) Oxidants and antioxidants in exercise. *J.Appl. Physiol.* **79**: 675–686.

Sen, C. K., Atalay, M., and Hänninen, O. (1994a) Exercise-induced oxidative stress: glutathione supplementation and deficiency. *J. Appl. Physiol.* **77**: 2177–2187.

Sen, C. K., Rahkila, P., and Hänninen, O. (1993) Glutathione metabolism in skeletal muscle derived cells of the L6 line. *Acta Physiol. Scand.* **148**: 21–26.

Sen, C. K., Rankinen, T., Väisänen, S., and Rauramaa, R. (1994b) Oxidative stress after human exercise: effect of N-acetylcysteine supplementation. *J. Appl. Physiol.* **76**: 2570–2577.

Shidlovskaya, T. E. (1985) Intensity of lipid peroxidation in tissues of hypokinetic rats. *Kosm. Biol. Aviakosm. Med.* **19**: 45–48.

Sibińska, E., Blaszczyk, J., Kowalczyk, P., Kędziora, J., and Lewicki, R. (1997) Research on the activity of Cu,Zn-SOD at the maximum height of physical strain among people of different levels of physical efficiency. *Wych. Fiz. Sport.* **3**: 65–70.

Sjödin, B., and Westing, Y. H. (1990) Changes in plasma concentration of hypoxanthine and uric acid in man with short-distance running at various intensities. *Acta Physiol. Scand.* **148**: 21–26.

Smirnov, V. V., and Potapov, P. P. (1981) Activity of succinate dehydrogenase and cytochrome oxidase in hypokinetic rats. *Kosm. Biol. Aviakosm. Med.* **15**: 69–71.

Somani, S. M. (1994) Influence of exercise-induced stress on the central nervous system. In *Exercise and Oxygen Toxicity*, edited by C. K. Sen, L. Packer, and O. Hänninen, Elsevier: Amsterdam, pp. 463–479.

Somani, S. M., and Husain, K. (1996) Exercise training alters kinetics of antioxidant enzymes in rat tissue. *Biochem. Mol. Biol. Int.* **38**: 587–595.

Sumida, S., Tanaka, K., Kitao, H., and Nakadomo, F. (1989) Exercise-induced lipid peroxidation and leakage of enzymes before and after vitamin E supplementation. *Int. J. Biochem.* **21**: 835–838.

Taneyeva, G. V., Potapovich, G. M., Voloshko, N. A., and Uteshev, A. B. (1979) Dynamics of erythrocyte count, hemoglobin, and catalase activity in rat blood in hypokinesia, muscular activity and restoration. *Izv. Akad. Nauk Kaz. SSR, Ser. Biol.* **1**: 71–74.

Tessier, F., Hida, H., Favier, A., and Marconnet, P. (1995b) Muscle GSH-Px activity after prolonged exercise, training, and selenium supplementation. *Biol. Trace Elem. Res.* **47**: 279–285.

Tessier, F., Margaritis, I., Richard, M. J., Moynot, C., and Marconnet, P. (1995a) Selenium and training effects on the glutathione system in response to exercise and training, and aerobic performance. *Med. Sci. Sports Exerc.* **27**: 390–396.

Toskulkao, C., and Glinsukon, T. (1996) Endurance exercise and muscle damage: relationship to lipid peroxidation and scavenging enzymes in short and long distance runners. *Jpn. J. Phys. Fitness Sports Med.* **45**: 63–70.

Venditti, P., and Di Meo, S. (1996) Antioxidants, tissue damage, and endurance in trained and untrained young male rats. *Arch. Biochem. Biophys.* **331**: 63–68.

Venditti, P., and Di Meo, S. (1997) Effect of training on antioxidant capacity, tissue damage, and endurance of adult male rats. *Int. J. Sports Med.* **18**: 497–502.

Viguie, C. A., Frei, B., Shigenaga, M. K., Ames, B. N., Packer, L., and Brooks, G. A. (1990) Oxidant stress in human beings during consecutive days of exercise. *Med. Sci. Sports Exerc.* 22:86S.

Viguie, C. A., Frei, B., Shigenaga, M. K., Ames, B. N., Packer, L., and Brooks, G. A. (1993) Antioxidant status and indexes of oxidative stress during consecutive days of exercise. *J. Appl. Physiol.* **75**: 566–572.

Warren, J. A., Jenkins, R. R., Packer, L., Witt, E. H., and Armstrong, P. B. (1992) Elevated muscle vitamin E does not attenuate eccentric exercise-induced muscle injury. *J. Appl. Physiol.* **72**: 2168–2175.

Witt, E. H., Reznick, A. Z., Viguie, C. A., Stark-Reed, P., and Packer, L. (1992) Exercise, oxidative damage and effects of antioxidant manipulation. *J. Nutr.* **122**: 766–773.

Zezerov, A. E., Ivanova, S. M., Morukov, B. V., and Ushakov, A. S. (1989) Lipid peroxidation in the human blood during a 120-day period of anti-orthostatic hypokinesia. *Kosm. Biol. Aviakosm. Med.* **23**: 28–33.

CHAPTER 6

Water Immersion Deconditioning in Medicine

Andrzej Wiecek, Michal Nowicki, and Franciszek Kokot

*Department of Nephrology, Endocrinology, and Metabolic Diseases,
Silesian University School of Medicine, Katowice, Poland*

> Give me health and a day and I will
> make the pomp of emperors ridiculous.
>
> *Emerson*

INTRODUCTION

Hydrotherapy, one of the oldest of the therapeutic methods, has been used for more than 20 centuries (Krizek, 1963). However, it was not until 1847 that scientific examination of the water immersion (WI) model was begun (Hartshorne, 1847). At that time Hartshorne recognized the diuretic response to immersion and proposed a mechanism for the diuresis; that is, that the heart posesses volume receptors capable of sensing the fullness of the blood stream as modified by WI (Hartshorne, 1847). Although Bazett et al. (1924) were the pioneers of systematic examination of the influence of WI on the human body, it was the advent of the space program that gave a new impetus to the use of WI as a nonaggressive investigative tool (Norsk and Epstein, 1991). Studies performed on astronauts revealed a significant hypovolemia and decrease in total body water, a consequence of the headward redistribution of body fluids that takes place in a gravity-free environment (Graveline and McCally, 1962; Leach, 1987; Leach and Rambaut, 1977; Lutwak et al., 1969). Because some of the responses to WI mimic some of those to weightlessness deconditioning, the WI model has attracted wide interest as a means for studying the influence of weightlessness on hemodynamic, metabolic, and nervous system processes on Earth.

In human studies in which WI is used as an analog of weightlessness it is necessary to maintain the water bath temperature at 34.5°C (94.1°F) to assure body thermoneutrality. Alteration of bath temperature significantly influences the physiological (especially the cardiovascular) responses to immersion. Weston et al. (1987) characterized the cardiovascular response to WI at different temperatures. They found that cardiac output rose progressively to reach 12% at high water temperature [39°C (102.2°F)], and that circulatory vascular peripheral resistance decreased progressively with increasing bath temperature. At 39°C (102.2°F) tachycardia occurs and contributes to the markedly augmented cardiac output. Finally, increasing the water temperature diminishes natriuresis. These responses suggested the importance of maintaining a neutral water temperature to avoid confounding influences on cardiovascular and renal hemodynamics and excretory function. Special thermal homeostatic controllers are used to maintain a constant thermoneutral water temperature [34–35°C (93.2–95°F)] (Peterson et al., 1987) throughout the immersion protocol.

Utilization of WI in studies of humans was established in the early 1900s. At present there are no standard or uniform experimental procedures. Several modifications of WI procedures have been proposed because the testing procedures used in WI studies have varied markedly. For example, it is important that the body be immersed up to the neck and that a semirecumbent body position be maintained. In this position the hydrostatic pressure exerted on the body redistributes blood and body fluids upward toward volume receptors. Some investigators have used a special table installed in the water baths that can be used to tilt the body forward, backward, and laterally. Several highly sophisticated immersion facilities have also been introduced for monitoring physiological reactions (Koepke and DiBona, 1987).

Immersion media vary, but tap water is usually used; exceptions include various solutions of sodium chloride (Graybiel and Clark, 1961; Howard et al., 1967). Ish-Shalom and Better (1984) carried out a WI study in the extremely hypertonic water of the Dead Sea and concluded that the saline bath induced a more profound effect on circulatory homeostasis than did tap water. Finally, Webb and Annis (1966) used a silicon fluid as medium to reduce skin maceration during prolonged immersion.

PHYSIOLOGICAL ALTERATIONS INDUCED BY WATER IMMERSION

Hemodynamic Changes

In the first 20–30 min of WI plasma volume increases by 8.3% (Khosla and DuBois, 1981) to 9% (McCally, 1964). There are some differences between measured and calculated changes of plasma volumes, but the differences are probably a result of variable changes in red blood cell volume during WI.

Following the highest increase in plasma volume after about 20 min of WI, there is a subsequent linear decrease of plasma volume (Greenleaf, 1984). This increase in plasma volume is a result of marked redistribution of body fluids, especially from the interstitial space, with a relative increase in central blood volume. The central hemodynamic alterations induced by WI are identical to those obtained by infusion of 2 liters of saline solution during 120 min (Levinson et al., 1977). The magnitude of these hemodynamic effects is dependent on the specific weight and temperature of the immersion fluid used, on the depth of the bath, and on the duration of the WI (Aborelius et al., 1972; Epstein, 1976; Greenleaf, 1984). As a consequence of increased mechanical pressure on tissues and of abdominal compression induced by WI, there is an isotonic shift of interstitial fluid into the vascular space, at least during the first hour of WI (Greenleaf et al., 1980, 1981). Hyponatremia is not a consistent finding during WI (Epstein et al., 1973, 1981). During WI the mean cardiac output increases by 32% and mean stroke volume by 35% (Aborelius et al., 1972); both the right atrial and pulmonary arterial transmural pressure gradients increase. Systemic vascular resistance increases by about 35% (Aborelius et al., 1972; Echt et al., 1974).

In healthy subjects WI results in an increase of heart volume by 180 ± 62 ml (Lange et al., 1974). The increase in cardiac index is dependent on the age of the subjects; WI increased the cardiac output of healthy elderly subjects by 59% and of young subjects by only 22% (Thames, 1977).

There are discrepancies in changes in blood pressure during WI. It had been suggested that systemic blood pressure was unchanged during WI (Epstein, 1978); however, data from more recent studies (Chudek et al., 1997; Norsk et al., 1985, 1986) indicate significant decreases in blood pressure. A greater decrease in blood pressure was observed in hypertensive than in normotensive subjects (Coruzzi et al., 1985b).

The increase of central blood volume is accompanied by decreases of interstitial fluid volume and plasma osmolality. The exact mechanism of WI-induced hemodilution is not clear. It was calculated that the leg fluid volume of healthy subjects decreased by 192 ± 20 ml during WI (Tajima et al., 1989). More recent data suggest that this decrease is caused by a shift of fluid not only from the interstitial space, but also from the intracellular fluid compartment into the vascular space (Hinghofer-Szalkay et al., 1987; Miki et al., 1987). An important role is also played by the fluid shifts in the capillary bed of the leg (Johansen et al., 1995).

Respiratory Changes

Water immersion induces upward movement of the diaphragm and causes depressed respiratory function. It decreases total lung capacity by 3–10%, vital capacity by 3–5%, and functional residual capacity by 40% (Prefaut et al., 1979); pulmonary compliance remains unchanged (Boehm and Ekert, 1938; Lundgreen, 1984). Reduction of total lung capacity is mainly a result of increased hydrostatic pressure on the chest and increased intrathoracic blood volume. WI also induces a more uniform redistribution of the ventilation/perfusion ($\dot{Q}/\dot{V}$) ratio in the lungs (Lundgreen, 1984).

In spite of the significant increase that WI causes in the intravascular space of the pulmonary capillaries, neither tissue nor capillary blood volume changes during WI (Begin et al., 1976).

The fact that vital capacity does not change suggests that the increase of central blood volume during WI does not induce a shift of fluid into lung interstitial tissue (Begin et al., 1976). By increasing diuresis, WI prevents pulmonary overhydration.

Renal Changes

Since WI causes central volume expansion, some compensatory mechanisms counteracting these hemodynamic alterations may be expected. In fact, WI induces a significant diuresis, natriuresis, and kaliuresis. In 1951 Cargill, Sellers, and Shure first reported that normal subjects immersed in water in the upright position to heart level showed an increase in glomerular filtration rate (GFR), and not a decrease as had been observed during the upright position in air. Recent data suggest that GFR (assessed by inulin clearance) does not change during WI, whereas renal blood flow increases significantly by about 15% (Coruzzi et al., 1986; Coruzzi et al., 1984; Myers et al., 1988). The magnitude of these effects is dependent on the state of hydration and sodium–potassium balance (Nakamitsu et al., 1994); consequently there is a small but significant decline (by 2%) in the filtration fraction.

Intrarenal venous pressure (as an index of peritubular hydrostatic capillary pressure) increases owing to renal vasodilatation during the first hour of immersion; there is a further increment in the second hour. Analysis of the transglomerular dextran transport indicates that glomerular capillary pressure declines in response to WI (Myers et al., 1988). Consistently, calculated renal vascular resistance (RVR) decreases by 16% to 33% during WI (Coruzzi et al., 1988a; Nakamitsu et al., 1994).

The exact mechanism of WI-induced diuresis and natriuresis is complex. It seems that suppression of the renin–angiotensin–aldosterone (RAA) system (Coruzzi et al., 1984; Coruzzi et al., 1986; Myers et al., 1988), vasopressin secretion (Dutawa et al., 1987; Epstein, 1976; Harrison et al., 1986), and activity of the sympathetic nervous system (Epstein et al., 1985; O'Hare et al., 1986b), as well as stimulation of renal prostaglandin synthesis (Epstein et al., 1979; Nakamitsu et al., 1994) and secretion of natriuretic factors (Coruzzi et al., 1986; Epstein, 1992; Pandergast et al., 1987) contribute to the increased WI-induced excretion of water, sodium, and potassium by the kidneys.

As mentioned above, WI induces a significant increase in the central blood volume and, consequently, in renal blood flow. However, some evidence suggests that WI-induced natriuresis is a result of decreased reabsorption of sodium, both in the proximal and distal segments of the nephron, rather than of alterations in the filtered sodium load (Epstein et al., 1973; Epstein et al., 1975a; Vesely et al., 1995). Some possible mechanisms of WI-induced natriuresis are shown in Figure 6.1. Additionally, a recently discovered kaliuretic peptide (Vesely et al., 1995)—a 98-amino-acid fragment of an ANP prohormone released by WI—may participate in the WI-enhanced kaliuresis.

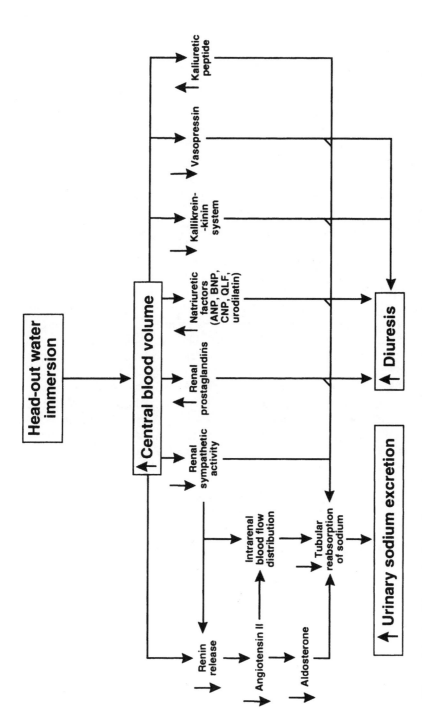

Figure 6.1 Possible mechanisms of water-immersion-induced increase of diuresis and natriuresis (ANP: atrial natriuretic peptide; BNP: brain natriuretic peptide; CNP: C-type natriuretic peptide; OLF: ouabain-like factor).

More recently Johansen et al. (1995) found that the decrease in colloid osmotic pressure during WI is due to fluid shifts in the capillary bed of the leg and may account for 25% of WI-induced natriuresis.

In addition to natriuresis and kaliuresis, WI induces a significant increase of calcium excretion by the kidneys (Coruzzi et al., 1993a), as well as of magnesium and bicarbonates (Behn et al., 1969; Brown et al., 1983; Lin and Hong, 1984). Phosphate and uric acid excretion by the kidneys are decreased during the first hour of WI, but increase subsequently (Brown et al., 1983; Epstein et al., 1976).

There are other important factors which may participate in the natriuretic response to WI. Coruzzi et al. (1989) found that the correlation between the natriuretic response and urodilatin was higher than that between the natriuretic response and atrial natriuretic peptide (ANP).

Endocrine Changes

Renin–angiotensin–aldosterone (RAA) system

It is generally agreed that WI induces a suppressive effect on the renin–angiotensin–aldosterone system (Coruzzi et al., 1985a; Epstein et al., 1975a; Kokot et al., 1989c; Kokot et al., 1983). There was a decline in plasma renin activity after 30 min of WI, and then a further decrease to 40–50% of the basal value after 1–2 hr of WI; after WI the activity level quickly returned to normal (Epstein et al., 1975b; Epstein and Saruta, 1971; Greenleaf, 1984).

Epstein et al. (1975b) studied the influence of WI on plasma aldosterone in a group of normal subjects during dietary sodium restriction; they found significant suppression of aldosterone beginning after 60 min, with a peak suppression of 34% of the control value after 210 min of WI. After discontinuation of WI there was a prompt return of the aldosteronemia to pre-study levels. The mechanism of WI-induced suppression of RAA is not clear. Perhaps, following the central hypervolemia, the right atrial volume receptors are stimulated with subsequent decreases in renal sympathetic nerve activity and renin secretion and an increase in ANP secretion (Epstein et al., 1975b; Gauer, 1978).

Increased delivery of sodium to the distal tubule (macula densa) may also participate in the pathogenesis of the suppression of renin secretion (Rabelink et al., 1989). The attenuation of WI-induced aldosteronemia parallels changes in plasma renin activity (Epstein and Saruta, 1971).

Atrial natriuretic peptide (ANP) and arginine vasopressin (AVP)

An increase in plasma ANP release may also play an important role in the pathogenesis of decreased renin secretion (Stasch et al., 1988). Immersion in thermoneutral water induces a significant decrease of plasma AVP concentration in healthy subjects; this effect may be observed after the first 30–60 min of immersion (Greenleaf et al., 1981; Epstein et al., 1981). The effect of WI on AVP secretion depends on the level of body hydration: the decrease in plasma AVP in dehydrated subjects (Greenleaf et al., 1983) is usually much greater than that in normovolemic subjects; but other investigators found no significant influence of WI on AVP or, on the contrary, even found an increase of vasopressin during WI (Greenleaf et al., 1983). The reason for such discrepancies may be the different hydration states of the subjects. The mechanism of the significant suppression of plasma AVP concentration is complex and not completely clear (Norsk and Epstein, 1988). But a decrease of AVP during WI is accounted for by a marked increase in aquaporin-2 in healthy subjects (Buemi et al., 2000).

Atrial peptides are also involved in the regulation of natriuresis and plasma volume during WI (Epstein, 1976; Gauer et al., 1970). Activation of stretch receptors located mainly in the right atrium is followed by an increased secretion of ANP (Epstein et al., 1975b; Gauer, 1978). During WI, central volemia increases and atrial filling is increased with subsequent stimulation of atrial receptors (Greenleaf et al., 1983; Greenleaf, 1984). This stimulation explains the increment of ANP during WI. Epstein et al. (1986a) showed that 3 hr of WI was followed by a two- to fourfold increase in plasma ANP. After completion of WI, plasma ANP declines rapidly and reaches preimmersion levels within 60 min (Epstein et al., 1986a).

Similar to its effect on AVP concentration, the hydration state of the subject may determine the magnitude of ANP secretion (Pendergast et al., 1987) because an attenuated response of ANP secretion during WI was found in dehydrated subjects (Claybaugh et al., 1986).

This response can also explain differences concerning WI-induced ANP secretion. For example, Kurosawa et al. (1988) reported that ANP did not increase significantly during WI; but the subjects underwent fluid restriction before WI and did not receive fluids during immersion.

The increase of ANP secretion is responsible for the increased natriuresis induced by WI. However, central blood volume expansion also induces many other hemodynamic, neural, and hormonal responses that might potentiate the renal response to this peptide. As a result, infusion of exogenous ANP at blood-level concentrations in subjects in air similar to those observed during WI induces a less pronounced natriuresis (60% of baseline values), in comparison with that induced in subjects in WI of 130% of baseline values (Anderson et al., 1987). Infusion of natriuretic doses of exogenous ANP into subjects in air is followed by simultaneous decreases of plasma volume and pulmonary wedge pressure (Cody et al., 1986; Henrich et al., 1986). Quite opposite physiologic effects occur during WI (Begin et al., 1976; Levinson et al., 1977; Norsk and Epstein, 1988). It would seem that the use of specific antagonists of ANP during WI may elucidate precisely the role of ANP for WI-induced natriuresis.

In parallel with the WI-induced increase of plasma ANP levels, there is an increase of urinary cyclic guanosine monophosphate (GMP) (Myers et al., 1988). This increase is consistent with the renal action of ANP, which may substantially contribute to the observed renal responses to WI (Huang et al., 1986; Myers et al., 1988). Urodilatin, a member of the natriuretic peptide family, is produced selectively by the kidneys. Nakamitsu et al. (1994) have found that urinary urodilatin is increased in parallel with ANP and c-GMP; they reported a higher correlation of the WI-induced natriuretic response with urodilatin than with ANP.

Drummer et al. (1991) found a dissociation between plasma ANP concentration and urinary sodium excretion during WI; they proposed that urodilatin may be the dominant regulator of natriuresis in subjects with increased central volemia induced by acute saline infusion. Water-immersion-induced increase of plasma ANP is also markedly reduced during the blockade of opioid receptors by naloxone (Widera et al., 1992).

The role of other natriuretic factors; for example, C-type natriuretic peptide (CNP), brain natriuretic peptide (BNP), and ouabain-like factor, in the natriuresis and diuresis induced by WI remains to be proven.

Catecholamines

Results concerning the influence of WI on plasma catecholamines are conflicting. Some data indicate that WI induced significant increases in plasma adrenaline and noradrenaline (Graveline et al., 1961), whereas others found significantly decreased plasma catecholamine levels (Davydova et al., 1981; O'Hare et al., 1986). Additionally, plasma dopamine was increased (Davydova et al., 1981) or did not change (O'Hare et al., 1986) during WI. These conflicting results seem to be mainly a result of differences in the hydration status and body position of the subjects, water temperature, and the coexistence of different stress factors during WI.

A high correlation between urinary dopamine and natriuresis induced by WI was also found (Coruzzi et al., 1989). Theoretically, and from experimental data, it follows that increased central blood volume is followed by a significant decrease in plasma and urinary catecholamines (DiBona, 1978; Karim et al., 1972). Plasma noradrenaline concentration decreased progressively during 4 hr of saline infusion in air (Epstein et al., 1983). Both immersion and saline infusion caused an increase in the plasma/urinary dopamine ratio (Coruzzi et al., 1989). A significant positive correlation was also found between the mean dopamine/noradrenaline ratio and mean urinary sodium excretion during WI, as well as during saline infusion (Krishna et al., 1983). These findings suggest that neurohormonal mechanisms are contributing to the natriuretic response to central hypervolemia. These mechanisms comprise a persistent sympathoadrenal suppression and a later (after at least 2 hr of WI) increase in dopamine activity (Grossman et al., 1992).

The natriuresis induced by WI is blunted by pretreatment with dopaminergic blockers (Coruzzi et al., 1989), which strongly indicates involvement of the dopaminergic system in the natriuretic response to WI.

Endogenous opioid peptides

Coruzzi et al. (1988b) reported that 2 hr of WI induce a significant increase in plasma methenkephalin and a significant suppression of plasma β-endorphin concentrations. As was shown by Widera et al. (1992), an increased secretion of opioids may be involved in the hormonal response to WI.

ACTH–cortisol axis

In the few studies concerning the ACTH–cortisol axis, WI had a suppressive effect in healthy individuals, as well as in patients with various pathological conditions (Grzeszczak et al., 1986; Ogihara et al., 1986). However, Epstein (1976) found no significant changes in plasma cortisol during WI in healthy subjects. Activation of low-pressure receptors located in the chest may suppress the ACTH–cortisol axis during WI (Mancia et al., 1979). The improvement in renal excretory function induced by WI may contribute to the reduction in plasma cortisol that is produced by WI (Guyton et al., 1984).

Prostaglandins (PG)

The significant increase of urinary PGE excretion during WI (observed after 2 hr of WI) also occurred after pretreatment with PG synthesis inhibitors such as indo-methacin (Epstein et al., 1979). Although administration of indomethacin attenuates the augmentation of PG synthesis during WI, it does not impair the natriuresis. The physiological relationship between the renin-angiotensin system and synthesis of renal PG is dissociated during WI (Epstein et al., 1980). Epstein et al. (1989) have suggested that WI-induced central volume expansion is the main factor influencing renal PG excretion. Preliminary observations suggest that PGI2 might contribute to the natriuretic and diuretic response induced by WI (Rabelink et al., 1991).

Erythropoietin

Two-hour WI increases plasma erythropoietin levels both in healthy subjects and in patients with essential hypertension (Chudek et al., 1997); participation of the renin–angiotensin system and ANP in the WI-induced increase in erythropoietin secretion seems to be unlikely in both normotensives and hypertensives.

Prolactin

Fiore et al. (1987) found no significant changes in prolactinemia during hypervolemia induced by WI.

Other hormones

Secretion of endothelins 1 to 3 increases during WI in parallel with catecholamines, both in healthy subjects and in patients with complicated liver cirrhosis (Gulberg and Gerbes, 1995).

A kaliuretic peptide which is a potent stimulator of both potassium and water excretion by the kidneys was discovered recently (Vesely et al., 1995); WI increases release of this kaliuretic peptide, especially in patients with liver cirrhosis (Vesely et al., 1996).

Kallikrein–kinin system

WI significantly suppresses the kallikrein–kinin system (O'Hare et al., 1986).

PERSPECTIVES ON THE CLINICAL APPLICATION OF WATER IMMERSION

Edemata of Different Origins

Physiological responses to water immersion are characterized mainly by increased diuresis and natriuresis. Therefore it seems reasonable to use WI as an important therapeutic maneuver in patients with edema of different etiologies; for example, in the treatment of overhydration in patients with liver cirrhosis, preeclampsia, nephrotic syndrome, and idiopathic edema. These and others are discussed below.

Liver Cirrhosis

Immersion has been used both as an investigative tool in the study of water–electrolyte abnormalities in liver cirrhosis, and as a therapeutic procedure in edematous patients (Bichet et al., 1983; Epstein et al., 1985; Gerbes et al., 1993). Hemodynamic monitoring (Swan-Ganz catheter) has been used throughout WI to determine changes in cardiac output, right-atrial and pulmonary-wedge pressures, and systemic vascular resistance (Bichet et al., 1983).

It is important to emphasize that cirrhotic patients with liver cirrhosis exhibit heterogeneous responses to natremia and AVP secretion (Epstein et al., 1984). In spite of these differences, WI can be used as a adjuvant method for treatment of edema in liver cirrhosis in addition to diuretic therapy. Additional use of spironolactone (aldactone) may augment the natriuretic and diuretic effect of WI (Gerbes et al., 1993). Despite a considerable increase in effective blood volume in patients with liver cirrhosis, WI does not restore the impaired renal function in these patients.

Nephrotic Syndrome

Berlyne et al. (1981) first demonstrated the possibility of using WI to examine renal sodium and water handling in patients with the nephrotic syndrome. Immersion induced a marked natriuresis and diuresis and led to significant weight loss. A concomitant decrease of plasma aldosterone was also found in these patients (Kokot, 1989c; O'Hare et al., 1988). The pathophysiological role of ANP in renal sodium handling during WI in nephrotic patients has been assessed (Peterson et al., 1988). These patients are characterized by a reduced natriuretic and diuretic response to WI, in comparison with healthy controls, in spite of a markedly greater increment in plasma ANP levels (Peterson et al., 1988). These results suggest a reduced sensitivity of the collecting tubules to the natriuretic action of ANP in nephrotic patients, which may contribute to the development of their edema. In light of these results it seems that WI may serve as an additional therapeutic maneuver in nephrotic patients.

Preeclampsia

Pregnancy is characterized by an increase in circulating plasma volume; this increase is less pronounced in women with preeclampsia. When immersion-induced endocrine alterations were examined in healthy pregnant women and in women with mild to moderate late pregnancy preeclampsia, it was shown that WI induced a prompt fall of mean arterial blood pressure which was accompanied by decreases of plasma renin activity and plasma aldosterone (Ulman-Doniec et al., 1987). In contrast to non-pregnant women, healthy pregnant women and women with preeclampsia showed a significantly attenuated WI-induced increase in plasma ANP levels. Despite these differences in the hormonal reaction patterns, the WI-induced diuresis was similar in all groups. These results suggest that factors other than ANP may be involved in WI-induced enhanced diuresis.

Arterial Hypertension

Water immersion induces a significantly greater decline in the blood pressure of patients with essential hypertension than does bed rest (Henry, 1995). Regardless of the etiology of the hypertension (essential, renal, or renovascular), WI induces a significant decrease in plasma renin activity and AVP concentration, but a significant increase in ANP which was quantitatively different from that in normotensive subjects (Epstein et al., 1986b; Larochelle et al., 1994). Immersion-induced endocrine alterations are not related to either the severity of or the etiology of hypertension (Coruzzi et al., 1985a; Epstein et al., 1986b). Immersion-induced reduction in blood pressure was not related to the above-mentioned endocrine alterations (Coruzzi et al., 1985a). Therefore, it seems that factors other than decreases in plasma renin activity and aldosterone and AVP concentrations are mediating the WI-induced hypotension (Kokot et al., 1989e). Findings from WI studies performed in hypertensive patients after naloxone administration suggest that opioid receptors play an important role in the regulation of ANP secretion both in normotensive subjects and in patients with essential hypertension (Widera et al., 1992). As mentioned previously, Coruzzi et al. (1989) suggested that the dopaminergic system is a major determinant of the exaggerated WI-induced natriuresis in patients with essential hypertension. It should be stressed that WI also induces marked supression of peripheral plasma renin activity and mean arterial pressure in patients with reno-vascular hypertension (Coruzzi et al., 1985a).

Calcium antagonists given prior to WI may increase natriuresis (Coruzzi et al., 1993b).

Acute and Chronic Renal Failure

Patients with *acute renal failure* at the oliguric/anuric phase are characterized by markedly elevated ANP levels and a normal physiological regulatory mechanism for

ANP secretion, although by a reduced response of ANP release triggered by central volume expansion (Kokot et al., 1989, Kokot et al., 1990). Patients with *chronic and acute renal failure* are also characterized during WI by a similar but quantitatively different response in plasma renin activity, aldosterone, and AVP secretion when compared with normal subjects (Kokot et al., 1989c).

Patients with acute or chronic renal failure show a greater increase in plasma volume during WI than do healthy subjects (Kokot et al., 1989c), which seems to be a result of the impaired excretory function of the kidneys.

Kidney Transplant Patients

In spite of the lack of renal innervation, patients with a transplanted kidney show significant declines in plasma renin activity and in plasma aldosterone level and a natriuretic response to WI that is similar to that of healthy subjects (Kokot et al., 1989b), indicating that intact renal nerves are not mandatory for a normal renal response to WI in humans (Rabelink et al., 1993). We have found that patients with kidney transplants are characterized by a reduced response of ANP secretion to central hypervolemia (Kokot et al., 1989b); moreover, the kind of immunosupressive therapy that is used seems to play a minor role in the response of renin, AVP, and ANP secretion to WI.

Heart Transplant Patients

Immersion can be an important investigative tool in cardiac transplant recipients. Myers et al. (1988) and Kokot et al. (1989d) found that these transplant recipients are characterized by a normal response of ANP secretion to WI-induced hypervolemia, and they show WI-induced natriuresis and diuresis that are similar to those of healthy subjects. Immersion can be also used to elucidate the role of cardiac denervation in volume homeostasis.

Endocrine Disorders

Diabetes mellitus

Conflicting results have been obtained from WI studies of volume regulation in diabetic patients. Liebermann et al. (1991) and O'Hare et al. (1989) found that ANP levels were higher in diabetics than in controls, and that during WI there was exaggerated ANP secretion. In spite of elevated ANP levels, diabetic patients show a reduced natriuretic response to WI (Liebermann et al., 1991; O'Hare et al., 1988, 1989) suggesting kidney resistance to ANP. Following WI, 18 diabetic patients had significantly lower ANP secretion than normals (Kokot et al., 1989a). Given the WI reduction in ANP secretion in diabetic patients, WI-induced diuresis was comparable to that in healthy subjects (Liebermann et al., 1991). These results suggest that factors other than ANP are operative in the mechanism of WI-induced natriuresis and diuresis in diabetic patients.

Primary aldosteronism

The saline infusion test is widely used for differential diagnosis of patients with primary aldosteronism and in other hypertensive patients without excess mineralo-corticoid (Weiberger et al., 1979). Coruzzi et al. (1991) used WI to differentiate aldosterone-producing adenomas from idiopathic hyperaldosteronism; they concluded that WI is a suitable method for differentiating these two forms of primary aldosteronism.

In contrast to its use in differential diagnosis of primary aldosteronism, WI was of no value in the diagnosis of pheochromocytoma (Coruzzi et al., 1992).

CONCLUSIONS AND FUTURE PERSPECTIVES

In the last two decades there has been increasing interest in the adaptive physio-logical responses to water immersion. This interest stems from the use of WI to simulate the spaceflight environment for studying physiological responses to that environment, as well as for studying volume and water-electrolyte abnormalities over a wide range of human pathological settings. As a result, WI is now recognized not only as a diagnostic tool, but also as a treatment for decompensated liver cirrhosis (Epstein et al., 1984, 1985), nephrotic syndrome (Berlyne et al., 1981; Peterson et al., 1988), preeclampsia (Kokot et al., 1983; Łukan-Doniec et al., 1987), and some forms of arterial hypertension (Coruzzi et al., 1985b, 1991; Epstein et al., 1986b). It can be expected that applications of the water-immersion technique will gain further scientific, diagnostic, and therapeutic relevance.

REFERENCES

Aborelius, M., Balldin, U. I., and Lilja, B. (1972) Haemodynamic changes in man during immersion with the head above water. *Aerospace Med.* **43**: 592–598.

Anderson, J. V., Donckier, J., Payne, N. N., Beacham, J., Slater, J. D. H., and Bloom, S. R. (1987) Atrial natriuretic peptide: evidence of action as a natriuretic hormone at physiological plasma concentrations in man. *Clin. Sci.* **72**: 305–312.

Bazett, H. C., Thurlow, S., Crowell, C., and Stewert, W. (1924) Studies on the effects of baths on man: the diuresis caused by warm bath, together with some observations on urinary tides. *Am. J. Physiol.* **70**: 430–452.

Begin, R., Epstein, M., Sackner, M. A., Levinson, R., Dougherty, R., and Duncan, D. (1976) Effects of water immersion to the neck in pulmonary circulation and tissue volume in man. *J Appl Physiol.* **40**: 293–299.

Behn, C., Gauer, O. H., Kirsch, K., and Eckert, P. (1969) Effects of sustained intrathoracic vascular distension on body fluid distrubution and renal excretion in man. *Pfluegers*

Archiv. **313**: 123–136.

Berlyne, G. M., Sutton, J., Brown, C., Feinroth, M. V., Feinroth, M., Adler, A. J., and Friedman, E. A. (1981) Renal salt and water handling in water immersion in the nephrotic syndrome. *Clin. Sci.* **61**: 605–610.

Bichet, D. G., Groves, B. M., and Schrier, R. W. (1983) Mechanisms of improvement of water and sodium excretion by immersion in decompensated cirrhotic patients. *Kidney Int.* **24**: 788–794.

Boehm, G., and Ekert, F. (1938) Appreciable x-ray evidence of the influence of daily or therapeutic baths on the central circulatory organs in healthy subjects. *Dtsch. Arch. Klin. Med.* **182**: 598–610.

Brown, C., Sutton, J. V., Adler, A., Feinroth, M. V., Feinroth, M., Friedman, E. A., and Berlyne, G. M. (1983) Renal calcium and magnesium handling in water immersion in nephrotic patients. *Nephron* **33**: 17–20.

Buemi, M., Corica, F., DiPasquale, G., Aloisi, C., Sofi, M., Casuscelli, T., Floccari, F., Senatore, M., Corsonello, A., Frisina, N. (2000) Water immersion increases urinary excretion of aquaporin-2 in healthy humans. *Nephron* **85**: 20–26.

Cargill, W. H., Sellers, S., and Shure, M. (1951) Induced variations in glomerular filtration rate and the urinary excretion of water and chloride. *Am. J. Med.* **11**: 239–240.

Chudek, J., Wicek, A., and Kokot, F. (1997) Influence of water immersion on plasma erythropoietin concentration in patients with essential hypertension. *Kidney Blood Press. Res.* **20**: 406–410.

Claybaugh, J. R., Pendergast, D. R., Davis, J. E., Akiba, C., Pazik, M., and Hong, S. K. (1986) Fluid conservation in athletes: responses to water intake, supine posture, and immersion. *J. Appl. Physiol.* **61**: 7–15.

Cody, R. J., Atlas, S. A., Laragh, J. H., Kubo, S. H., Covit, A. B., Ryman, K. S., Saknovich, A., Pondolfino, K., Clark, M., Camargo, M. J. F., Scarborough, R. M., and Lewicki, J. A. (1986) Atrial natriuretic factor in normal subjects and heart failure patients. *J. Clin. Invest.* **78**: 1362–1374, .

Coruzzi, P., Biggi, A., Musiari, L., Coriati, R., Mossini, G. L., Gueri, A., and Novarini, A. (1993a) Calcium and sodium handling during volume expansion in essential hypertension. *Metabolism* **42**: 1331–1335.

Coruzzi, P., Biggi, A., Musiari, L., Ravanetti, C., and Novarini, A. (1985a) Renin-aldosterone system suppresssion during water immersion in renovascular hypertension. *Clin. Sci.* **68**: 609–612.

Coruzzi, P., Biggi, A., Musiari, L., Ravanetti, C., and Novarini, A. (1986) Renal hemodynamics and natriuresis during water immersion in normal humans. *Pfluegers Arch.* **407**: 638–642.

Coruzzi, P., Musiari, L., Biggi, A., Carra, N., Panzali, A. F., and Novarini A. (1991) A new diagnostic test for primary aldosteronism. *Am. J. Hypertens.* **4**: 694–699.

Coruzzi, P., Musiari, L., Biggi, A., Mossini, G. L., and Novarini, A. (1992) Renin-angiotensin system unresponsiveness in pheochromocytoma. *J. Human Hypertens.* **6**: 239–241.

Coruzzi, P., Musiari, L., Biggi, A., Ravanetti, C., Vallisa, D., Montanari, A., and Novarini, A. (1988a) Role of renal hemodynamics in the exaggerated natriuresis of essential hypertension. *Kidney Int.* **33**: 875–880.

Coruzzi, P., Musiari, L., Mossini, G. L., and Novarini, A. (1993b) Regulation of sodium excretion in human hypertension: long-term effects of calcium antagonist and angiotensin converting enzyme inhibitor. *J. Cardiovasc. Pharmacol.* **21**: 920–925.

Coruzzi, P. A., Novarini, A., Biggi, A., Lazzeroni, E., Musiari, L., Ravanetti, C., Tagliavini, S., and Borghetti, A. (1985b) Low pressure receptor activity and exaggerated natriuresis in essential hypertension. *Nephron* **40**: 309–315.

Coruzzi, P., Novarini, A., Musiari, L., Ravanetti, C., Ghielmi, S., Rodella, A., and Montanari, A. (1989) The antinatriuretic effect of dopaminergic blockade during volume expansion is independent of circulating atrial natriuretic factor. *Clin. Sci.* **77**: 479–484.

Coruzzi, P., Novarini, A., Musiari, L., Rossi, E., and Borghetti, A. (1984) Effects of central hypervolemia by water immersion on renin-aldosterone system and ACTH-cortisol axis in hemodialyzed patients. *Nephron* **36**: 238–241.

Coruzzi, P., Ravanetti, C., Musiari, L., Biggi, A., Vascovi, P. P., and Novarini, A. (1988b) Circulating opioid peptides during water immersion in normal man. *Clin. Sci.* **74**: 133–136.

Davydova, A. A., Tigranyan, R. A., and Shulzhenko, E. B. (1981) The sympatho-adrenal system in man in water immersion. *Kosm. Biol. Aviakosm. Med.* **15**: 30–34.

DiBona, G. F. (1978) Neural control of renal tubular sodium reabsorption in the dog. *Fed. Proc.* **37**: 1214–1217.

Drummer, C., Fiedler, F., Konig, A., and Gerzer, R. (1991) Urodilatin, a kidney-derived natriuretic factor, is excreted with a circadian rhythm and is stimulated by saline infusion in man. *J. Am. Soc. Nephrol.* **1**: 1109–1113.

Dutawa, J., Kokot, F., and Grzeszczak, W. (1987) Einfluss der Wasserimmersion auf die Plasmareninaktivitat, den Vasopressin-, und Aldosteronspiegel bei Diabetikern. *Z. Ges. Inn. Med.* **42**: 298–302.

Echt, M., Lange, L., and Gauer, O. H. (1974) Changes of peripheral venous tone and central transmural venous pressure during water immersion in a thermo-neutral bath. *Pfluegers Arch.* **352**: 211–217.

Epstein, M. (1976) Cardiovascular and renal effects of water immersion in man: application of the model in the assessment of volume homeostasis. *Circ. Res.* **39**: 619–628.

Epstein, M. (1978) Renal effects of head-out water immersion in man: implications for an understanding of volume homeostasis. *Physiol. Rev.* **58**: 529–581.

Epstein, M. (1992) Renal effects of head-out water immersion in humans: a 15-year update. *Physiol. Rev.* **72**: 563–621.

Epstein, M., Johnson, G., and Denunzio, A. G. (1983) Effects of water immersion on plasma catecholamines in normal humans. *J. Appl. Physiol.* **54**: 244–248.

Epstein, M., Katsikas, J. L., and Duncan, D. C. (1973) Role of mineralocorticoids in the natriuresis of water immersion in normal man. *Circ. Res.* **32**: 228–236.

Epstein, M., Larios, O., and Johnson, G. (1985) Effects of water immersion on plasma catecholamines in decompensated cirrhosis. *Miner. Electrolyte Metab.* **11**: 25–34.

Epstein, M., Lifschitz, R., and Haber, E. (1980) Dissociation of renin-aldosterone and renal prostaglandin E during volume expansion induced by immersion in normal man. *Clin. Sci.* **59**: 55–62.

Epstein, M., Lifschitz, M., Hoffman, D. S., and Stein, J. H. (1979) Relationship between renal prostaglandin E and renal sodium handling during water immersion in normal man. *Circ. Res.* **45**: 71–80.

Epstein, M., Loutzenhiser, R. D., Friedland, E., Aceto, R. M., Camargo, R. J. F., and Atlas, S. A. (1986a) Increases in circulating atrial natriuretic factor during immersion-induced central hypervolemia in normal humans. *J. Hypertens.* **4**(Suppl. 2): S93–S99.

Epstein, M., Loutzenhiser, R., and Levinson, R. (1986b) Spectrum of deranged sodium homeostasis in essential hypertension. *Hypertension* **8**: 422–432.

Epstein, M., Norsk, P., and Loutzenhiser, R. (1989) Effects of water immersion on atrial natriuretic release in humans. *Am. J. Nephrol.* **9**: 1–9.

Epstein, M. Pins, D. S., Arrington, R., Denunzio, A. G., and Engstrom, R. (1975a) Comparison of water immersion and saline infusion as means of inducing volume expansion in man. *J. Appl. Physiol.* **39**: 66–70.

Epstein, M., Pins, D. S., Sandro, J., and Haber, E. (1975b) Suppression of plasma renin and plasma aldosterone during water immersion in normal man. *J. Clin. Endocrinol. Metab.* **41**: 618–625.

Epstein, M., Pins, D. S., Silvers, W., Loutzenhiser, R., Canterboury, J. M., and Reiss, E. (1976) Failure of water immersion to influence parathyroid hormone secretion and renal phosphate handling in normal man. *J. Lab. Clin. Med.* **87**: 218–226.

Epstein, M., Preston, S., and Weitzman, R. E. (1981) Isoosmotic central blood volume expansion suppresses plasma arginine vasopressin in normal man. *J. Clin. Endocrinol. Metab.* **52**: 256–262.

Epstein, M., and Saruta, T. (1971) Effect of water immersion on renin aldosterone and renal sodium handling in normal man. *J. Appl. Physiol.* **31**: 368–374.

Epstein, M., Weitzman, R. E., Preston, S., and Denunzio, A. G. (1984) Relationship between plasma arginine vasopressin and renal water handling in decompensated cirrhosis. *Miner. Electrolyte Metab.* **10**: 155–165.

Fiore, C. E., Foti, G., Benenati, R., Malatino, L. S., Grimaldi, D. R., and Guzzardi, F. (1987) Modification of PRA, aldosterone, prolactin, and parathyroid hormone serum levels by "head-out" water immersion. *Riv. Eur. Sci. Med. Farmacol.* **9**: 147–151.

Gauer, O. H. (1978) Mechanoreceptors in the intrathoracic circulation and plasma volume control. In *The Kidney in Liver Disease*, edited by M. Epstein, Elsevier: New York, pp. 13–17.

Gauer, O. H., Henry, J. P., and Behn, C. (1970) The regulation of extracellular fluid volume. *Annu. Rev. Physiol.* **32**: 547–595.

Gerbes, A. L., Pilz, A., Wernze, H., and Jungst, D. (1993) Renal sodium handling and neurohumoral systems in patients with cirrhosis in sitting posture: effects of spironolactone and water immersion. *Clin. Invest.* **71**: 894–897.

Graveline, D. E., Balke, B., McKenzie, R. E., and Hartman, B. (1961) Psychobiologic effects of water immersion induced hypodynamics. *Aerospace Med.* **32**: 387–397.

Graveline, D. E., and McCally, M. (1962) Body fluid distrubution: implications for zero gravity. *Aerospace Med.* **33**: 1281–1290.

Graybiel, A., and Clark, B. (1961) Symptoms resulting from prolonged immersion in water: the problem of zero G asthenia. *Aerospace Med.* **32**: 181–196.

Greenleaf, J. E. (1984) Physiological responses to prolonged bed rest and fluid immersion in man. *J. Appl. Physiol.* **57**: 619–635.

Greenleaf, J. E., Morse, J. T., Barnes, P. R., Silver, J., and Keil, L. C. (1983) Hypervolemia and plasma vasopressin response during water immersion in men. *J. Appl. Physiol.* **55**: 1688–1693.

Greenleaf, J. E., Shvartz, E., and Keil, L. C. (1981) Hemodilution, vasopressin suppression, and diuresis during water immersion in man. *Aviat. Space Environ. Med.* **52**: 329–336.

Greenleaf, J. E., Shvartz, E., Kravik, S., and Keil, L. C. (1980) Fluid shifts and endocrine responses during chair and water immersion in man. *J. Appl. Physiol.* **48**: 79–88.

Grossman, E., Goldstein, D. S., Hoffman, A., Wacks, I. R., and Epstein, M. (1992) Effects of water immersion on sympathoadrenal and dopa-dopamine systems in humans. *Am. J. Physiol. Regulatory Integrative Comp. Physiol.* **262**: R993–R999.

Grzeszczak, W., Kokot, F., and Wiecek, A. (1986) Effect of water immersion on serum ACTH and cortisol concentration in patients with acute renal failure and in healthy subjects. *Acta Med. Pol.* **27**: 109–116.

Gulberg, V., and Gerbes, A. L. (1995) Relation of endothelins to volume regulating neurohumoral systems in patients with cirrhosis of the liver. *Eur. J. Clin. Invest.* **25**: 893–898.

Guyton, A. C., Manning, R. D., Hale, J. E., Norman, E. A., Young, D. B., and Pan, Y. L. (1984) The pathogenic role of the kidney. *J. Cardiovasc. Pharmacol.* **6**: S151–S161.

Harrison, M. H., Keil, L. C., Wade, C. A., Silver, J. E,, Geelen, G., and Greenleaf, J. E. (1986) Effect of hydration on plasma volume and endocrine responses to water immersion. *J. Appl. Physiol.* **61**: 1410–1417.

Hartshorne, H. (1847) *Water versus Hydrotherapy or an Assay on Water and Its True Relations to Medicine.* L. Loyd and P. Smith Press: Philadelphia, PA.

Henrich, W. L., Walker, B. R., Handelman, W. A., Erickson, A. L., Arnold, P. E., and Schrier, R. W. (1986) Effects of angiotensin II on plasma natriuretic hormone and renal water excretion. *Kidney Int.* **30**: 503–508, .

Henry, J. P. (1995) Historical perspective of cardiorenal integration. *Clin. Exp. Pharmacol. Physiol.* **22**: 43–48.

Hinghofer-Szalkay, H., Harrison, M. H., and Greenleaf, J. E. (1987) Early fluid and protein shifts in men during water immersion. *Eur. J. Appl. Physiol.* **56**: 673–678.

Howard, P., Ernsting, J., Denison, D. M., Fryer, D. I., Glaister, D. H., and Byford, G. H. (1967) Effects of simulated weightlessness upon the cardiovascular system. *Aerospace Med.* **38**: 551–563.

Huang, C. L., Ives, H. E., and Cogan, M. G. (1986) In vivo evidence that cGMP is the second messenger for atrial natriuretic factor. *Proc. Natl. Acad. Sci. USA* **83**: 8015–1018.

Ish-Shalom, N., and Better, O. S. (1984) Volume regulation in man during neck-out immersion in a medium with high specific gravity (Dead Sea water). *Israel J. Med. Sci.* **20**: 109–112.

Johansen, L. B., Bie, P., Warberg, J., Christensen, N. J., Norsy, P. (1995) Role of hemodilution on renal responses to water immersion in humans. *Am. J. Physiol. Regulatory Integrative Comp. Physiol.* **269**: R1068 – R1076.

Karim, F., Kidd, C., Malpus, C. M., and Penna, P. E. (1972) The effects of stimulation of the left atrial receptors on sympathetic efferent nerve activity. *J. Physiol. (Lond.)* **227**: 243–260.

Khosla, S. S., and DuBois, A. B. (1981) Osmoregulation and interstitial fluid pressure changes in humans during water immersion. *J. Appl. Physiol.* **51**: 686 – 692.

Koepke, J. P., and DiBona, G. F. (1987) Blunted natriuresis to atrial natriuretic peptide in chronic sodium retaining disorders. *Am. J. Physiol. Renal Physiol.* **252**: F865–F871.

Kokot, F., Dulawa, J., Bar, A., Klin, M., Grzeszczak, W., and Darocha, Z. (1989a) Water-immersion-induced alterations of atrial natriuretic peptide, plasma renin activity, aldosterone and vasopressin in diabetic patients. *Contrib. Nephrol.* **73**: 102–110.

Kokot, F., Grzeszczak, W., and Wiecek, A. (1989) Water-immersion-induced alterations of atrial natriuretic peptide in patients with non-inflammatory acute renal failure. *Nephrol. Dial. Transplant.* **4**: 691–695.

Kokot, F., Grzeszczak, W., Wiecek, A., Żukowska-Szczechowska, E., Kuśmierski, S., and Szkodny, A. (1989b) Water-immersion-induced alterations of plasma atrial natriuretic peptide, plasma renin activity, plasma aldosterone, and vasopressin in kidney transplant recipients. *Transplant Proc.* **21**: 2052–2055.

Kokot, F., Grzeszczak, W., Żukowska-Szczechowska, E., and Wiecek A. (1989c) Water-immersion-induced alterations of plasma atrial natriuretic peptide and its relationship to the renin-angiotensin-aldosterone system and vasopressin secretion in acute and chronic renal failure. *Clin. Nephrol.* **31**: 247–252.

Kokot, F., Grzeszczak, W., Żukowska-Szczechowska, E., and Wiecek, A. (1990) Water-immersion-induced alterations of plasma vasopressin levels and activity of the renin-angiotensin-aldosterone system in noninflammatory acute renal failure and end-stage renal failure. *Int. Urol. Nephrol.* **22**: 285–293.

Kokot, F., Religa, Z., Pasyk, S., Wiecek, A., Frycz, J., Grzeszczak, W., Bochenek, A., and Dutawa, J. (1989d) Atrial natriuretic peptide secretion in heart transplant patients. *Int. J. Artif. Organs* **12**: 321–326.

Kokot, F., Ulman, J., and Cekański, A. (1983) Influence of head-out water immersion on plasma renin activity, aldosterone, vasopressin, and blood pressure in late pregnancy toxaemia. *Proc. Eur. Dial. Transpl. Assoc.* **20**: 557–561.

Kokot, F., Wiecek, A., Grzeszczak, W., Szczechowska, E., and Dulawa, J. (1989e) The water immersion model in nephrology. *Contrib. Nephrol.* **70**: 107–115.

Krishna, G. G., Danovitch, G. M., and Sowers, J. R. (1983) Catecholamine responses to central volume expansion produced by head-out water immersion and saline infusion. *J. Clin. Endocrinol. Metab.* **56**: 998–1002.

Krizek, V. (1963) History of balneotherapy. In *Medical Hydrology*, edited by S.Licht,

Waverly, pp. 131–159.

Kurosawa, T., Sakamoto, H., Katoh, Y., and Marumo, F. (1988) Atrial natriuretic peptide is only a minor diuretic factor in dehydrated subjects immersed to the neck in water. *Eur. J. Appl. Physiol.* **57**: 10–14.

Lange, L., Lange, S., Echt, M., and Gauer, O. H. (1974) Heart volume in relation to body posture and immersion in a thermo-neutral bath. *Pfluegers Arch.* **352**: 219–226.

Larochelle, P., Cusson, J. R., Du Souich, P., Hamet, P., and Schiffrin, E. L. (1994) Renal effects of immersion in essential hypertension. *Am. J. Hypertens.* **7**: 120–128.

Leach, C. S. (1987) Fluid control mechanisms in weightlessness. *Aviat. Space Environ. Med.* **58**(Suppl. 9): A74–A79.

Leach, C. S., and Rambaut, P. C. (1977) Biochemical responses of the Skylab crewmen: an overview. In *Biomedical Results From Skylab*, edited by R. S. Johnston and L. F. Dietlein, Washington, DC: NASA SP-377, pp. 204–215.

Levinson, R., Epstein, M., Sackner, M. A., and Begin, M. (1977) Comparison of the effects of water immersion and saline infusion on central haemodynamics in man. *Clin. Sci. Mol. Med.* **52**: 343–350.

Liebermann, J. S., Parra, L., Newton, L., Scandling, J. D., Loon, N., and Myers, B. D. (1991) Atrial natriuretic peptide response to changing plasma volume in diabetic nephropathy. *Diabetes* **40**: 893–901.

Lin, Y. C., and Hong, S. K. (1984) Physiology of water immersion. *Undersea Biomed. Res.* **1**: 139–147.

Lundgreen, C. E. G. (1984) Respiratory function during simulated wet dives. *Undersea Biomed. Res.* **1**: 139–147.

Lutwak, L., Whedon, G. D., Lachance, P. A., Reid, J. M., and Lipscomb, H. S. (1969) Mineral, electrolyte and nitrogen balance studies of the Gemini-VII fourteen-day orbital space flight. *J. Clin. Endocrinol. Metab.* **29**: 1140–1156.

McCally, M. (1964) Plasma volume response to water immersion: implications for space flight. *Aerospace Med.* **35**: 130–132.

Mancia, G., Donald, D. E., and Sheperd, J. T. (1979) Inhibition of adrenergic outflow to peripheral blood vessels by vagal afferents form the cardiopulmonary region in the dog. *Circ. Res.* **33**: 713–719.

Miki, K., Hajduczok, G., and Hong, S. K. (1987) Extracellular fluid and plasma volumes during water immersion in nephrectomised dogs. *Am. J. Physiol. Regulatory Integrative Comp. Physiol.* **252**: R972–R978.

Myers, B. D., Peterson, C., Molin, C., Tomlanovich, S. J., Newton, L. D., Nitkin, R., Sandler, H., and Murad, F. (1988) Role of cardiac atria in the human renal response to changing plasma volume. *Am. J. Physiol. Renal Physiol.* **254**: F562–F573.

Nakamitsu, S., Sagawa, S., Miki, K., Wada, F., Nagaya, K., Keil, L. C., Drummer, C., Gerzer, R., Greenleaf, J. E., and Hong, S. K.(1994) Effect of water temperature on diuresis-natriuresis: AVP, ANP, and urodilatin during immersion in men. *J. Appl. Physiol.* **77**: 1919–1925.

Norsk, P., Bonde-Petersen, F., and Warberg, J. (1985) Central venous pressure and plasma arginin vasopressin during water immersion in man. *Eur. J. Appl. Physiol.* **54**: 71–78.

Norsk, P., Bonde-Petersen, F., and Warberg, J. (1986) Arginine vasopressin, circulation, and kidney during graded water immersion in humans. *J. Appl. Physiol.* **61**: 565–574.

Norsk, P., and Epstein, M. (1988) Effects of water immersion on arginine vasopressin release in humans. *J. Appl. Physiol.* **64**: 1–10.

Norsk, P., and Epstein, M. (1991) Manned space flight and the kidney. *Am. J. Nephrol.* **11**: 81–97.

Ogihara, T., Shima, J., Hara, H., Tabuchi, Y., Hashizume, K., Nagano, M., Kajahira, K., Kangawa, K., Matsuo, H., and Kumahara, Y. (1986) Significant increase in plasma immunoreactive atrial natriuretic peptide concentration during head-out water immersion. *Life Sci.* **38**: 2413–2418.

O'Hare, J. P., Anderson, J. V., and Millar, N. D. (1989) Hormonal response to blood volume expansion in diabetic subjects with and without autonomic nephropathy. *Clin. Endocrinol.* **30**: 571–579.

O'Hare, J. P., Anderson, J. V., Millar, N. D., Bloom, S. R., and Corrall, R. J. (1988) The relationship of the renin-angiotensin-aldosterone system to atrial natriuretic peptide and the natriuresis of volume expansion in diabetics with and without proteinuria. *Postgrad. Med. J.* **64**(Suppl. 3): 35–38.

O'Hare, J. P., Dalton, N., and Roland, J. M. (1986) Plasma catecholamine levels during water immersion. *Horm. Metab. Res.* **18**: 713–716.

O'Hare, P., Bhoola, K., Chapman, I., Roland, J., and Corrall, R. (1986) Importance of circulating and urinary tissue kallikrein in the control of acute natriuresis and diuresis evoked by water immersion in man. *Adv. Exp. Med. Biol.* **198**: 225–232.

Pendergast, D. R., De Bold, A. J., Pazik, M., and Hong, S. K. (1987) Effects of head-out water immersion on plasma natriuretic factor in man. *Proc. Soc. Exp. Biol. Med.* **184**: 429–436.

Peterson, C., Madsen, B., Perlman, A., Chan, A. Y. M., and Myers, B. D. (1988) Atrial natriuretic peptide and the renal response to hypervolemia in nephrotic man. *Kidney Int.* **34**: 825–831.

Peterson, R. V., Benjamin, B. A., and Hurst, N. L. (1987) Effect of vagotomy and thoracic sympathectomy on responses of the monkey to water immersion. *J. Appl. Physiol.* **63**: 2476–2481.

Prefaut, C. F., DuBois, F., Russos, C., Amaral-Marques, R., Macklern, P. T., and Ruff, F. (1979) Influence of immersion to the neck in water on airways closure and distribution of perfusion in man. *Respir. Physiol.* **37**: 313–323.

Rabelink, T. J., Koomans, H. A., Boer, W. H., van Rijn, J., and Dorhout-Mees, E. J. (1989) Lithium clearance in water-immersion-induced natriuresis in humans. *J. Appl. Physiol.* **66**: 1744–1748.

Rabelink, T. J., Koomans, H. A., and Dorhout-Mees, E. J. (1991) Role of prostaglandins in the natriuresis of head-out water immersion in humans. *Clin. Sci.* **80**: 481–488.

Rabelink, T. J., van-Tilborg, K. A., Hene, R. J., and Koomans, H. A. (1993) Natriuretic response to head-out immersion in humans with recent kidney transplants. *Clin. Sci.* **85**: 471–477.

Stasch, J. P., Hirth, C., Kazda, S., and Neuser, D. (1988) The reduction of renin and aldosterone as a response to acute hypervolemia is blocked by a monoclonal antibody directly against atrial natriuretic peptides. *Life Sci.* **42**: 511–516.

Tajima, F., Ogata, H., Miki, K., Enishi, K., and Shiraki, K. (1989) Changes in limb volume during head-out water immersion in humans. *J. Univ. Occup. Environ. Health* **11**: 145–153.

Thames, M. D. (1977) Neutral control of renal function: contribution of cardiopulmonary baroreceptors to the control of the kidney. *Fed. Proc.* **37**: 1209–1213.

Ulman-Doniec, I., Kokot, F., Wannbach, G., and Drab, M. (1987) Water-immersion-induced endocrine alterations in women with EPH gestosis. *Clin. Nephrol.* **28**: 51–55.

Vesely, D. L., Norsk, P., Gower, Jr., W. R., Chiou, S., and Epstein, M. (1995) Release of kaliuretic peptide during immersion-induced central hypervolemia in healthy humans. *Proc. Soc. Exp. Biol. Med.* **209**: 20–26.

Vesely, D. L., Preston, R., Gower, Jr., W. R., Chiou, S., and Epstein, M. (1996) Increased release of kaliuretic peptide during immersion-induced central hypervolemia in cirrhotic humans. *Am. J. Nephrol.* **16**: 128–137.

Webb, P., and Annis, J. R. (1966) Silicone submersion – a feasibility study. *U.S. Naval Air Development Center*, Johnsville, PA, Report No. NADC-MR-6620, AD 645080.

Weiberger, M. H., Grim, C. E., and Hollifield, J. W. (1979) Primary aldosteronism: diagnosis, localisation, and treatment. *Ann. Intern. Med.* **90**: 386–395.

Weston, C. F. M., O'Hare, J. P., Evans, J. M., and Corrall, R. J. M. (1987) Haemodynamic changes in man during immersion in water at different temperatures. *Clin. Sci.* **73**: 613–616.

Widera, W., Kokot, F., and Wiecek, A. (1992) Do opioid receptors participate in the regulation of atrial natriuretic peptide secretion in hypertensive patients. *Clin. Nephrol.* **38**: 209–213.

CHAPTER 7

The Brittle Bones of Deconditioning

Helmut G. Hinghofer-Szalkay

Institute for Adaptive and Spaceflight Physiology,
Austrian Society for Aerospace Medicine, Graz, Austria

Better to hunt in fields, for health unbought,
than fee the doctor for a nauseous draught.
The wise, for cure, on exercise depend;
God never made his work, for man to mend.

John Dryden

INTRODUCTION

Bed rest (BR) deconditioning studies of healthy human subjects have provided a wealth of data on how the body normally reacts to reduced mechanical loading of the skeletal system. These studies were limited in duration, however, mostly for ethical reasons. Long-duration spaceflight offers an important alternative model; most missions have not yet lasted longer than 6 months, but some have already reached or exceeded 1 year. Future missions to Mars will last even longer, with at least 12 months of microgravity exposure for those traveling between Earth and Mars, and less than half of Earth's gravitational pull will be experienced during their stay there.

What have we learned about bone physiology and pathophysiology from simulated and real loss of gravitational acceleration, and what consequences ensue regarding the proper use of preventive measures against osteoporosis? Available knowledge will provide for application of novel therapeutic countermeasures which might revolutionize treatments for bone loss (Mundy et al., 1999; Vogel, 1999). This chapter first summarizes basic information about bone biomechanics, biochemistry, and physiology, and then presents their applied and clinical aspects, with emphasis on insights gained from research with human volunteers, astronauts, and patients.

Bone integrity is sustained by a cycle of constant formation of new bone and resorption of old bone. Mechanical stimuli act in a trophic fashion on bone tissue;

but how these forces are perceived, what the target cells are, how the sensors communicate messages into sensible cells, and by what pathways the cells finally respond are still unclear. But it seems that mechanisms mediating bone loss through disuse are similar in all forms and etiologies of osteoporosis, and that spaceflight— real and simulated—therefore provides valuable information on molecular and physiological mechanisms involved.

During prolonged BR the balance between bone formation and breakdown is disrupted and resorption predominates, resulting in bone loss and osteoporosis (Bloomfield, 1997; Fukuoka et al., 1994; LeBlanc et al., 1990, 1995; Nishimura et al., 1994; Vico et al., 1987). Osteoporosis is characterized by a parallel reduction in bone mineral and bone matrix so that bone content is decreased but its normal composition remains (Finkelstein et al., 1997). It is a common metabolic bone disease and represents a major health-care problem affecting up to 50% of all women and 25% of men over age 50, with the main consequence being hip and vertebral fractures (1.3 million per year in the U.S.). Medical treatment and long-term care of these patients cost many billions of dollars. One out of five patients will die within one year as a consequence of hip fracture. Osteoporosis can be caused by excessively increased bone resorption (low calcium availability, high calcium loss, hormonal disturbances), reduced bone formation (Nordin, 1997), or both.

About half the variance in bone density is stable because of an heredity-genetic baseline (Turner, 1999), but a large proportion of the nonheritable variance may be a result of life-style factors (Krall and Dawson-Hughes, 1993). The latter is the link to BR or immobilization: a significant life-style change that affects bone strength, fracture risk, and health and well-being. Prolonged BR, inactivity, or spaceflight are good models for investigations into the mechanisms of, and preventive strategies for, skeletal deconditioning and osteoporosis (Cowin, 1998; White, 1998). Research into its physiology, pathophysiology, diagnosis, and prevention is important for dedicated scientific, epidemiological, medical, and health-care workers.

Bone is one of the strongest biological materials on Earth because it contains organic materials that convey strength and stability, as well as minerals that contribute to stiffness—in a way similar to that of the steel rods and cement in reinforced concrete. Life on Earth has evolved under the constant influence of that ubiquitous force called gravity. When the first creatures left the sea about 400 million years ago, they had to evolve a strong weight-bearing skeletal system because their body mass was no longer supported by hydrostatic buoyancy (but water immersion can be employed as a model of deconditioning). On Earth, the largest forces affecting humans are usually those associated with gravity. On the other hand, any reduction of gravitational force also reduces the necessity for peak counter-force generation. In addition to longitudinal pressure, muscular force patterns are transmitted to bone as the supportive and power-distributing system; thus gravitational force directly and indirectly governs the trophic stimuli that bone continually receives. How this highly specialized bone tissue is capable of responding and adapting to these forces is the main topic of this chapter.

Osseal tissue has enormous capacity for growth, regeneration, and remodeling. The mechanism of osteoblast recruitment at the site of bone formation has not been fully elucidated, although the immediate environment of the cells plays a role by means of cell–matrix interactions. Matrix and cell surface proteoglycans are important for the control of cellular growth factors during chondrogenesis and osteogenesis. Integrins, which transduce signals from the extracellular matrix to the intracellular compartment, mediate the adhesion of osteoclasts during bone resorption. Vitamin D both upregulates integrin expression in mononucleated osteoclast precursors and stimulates their differentiation into osteoclasts, suggesting that integrins play a role during osteoclast differentiation (Boissy et al., 1998). However, the precise role of integrin molecules, individually and in concert, in bone–cell matrix interactions remains unclear.

To keep bone strong and flexible it is clear that the rigidity of the skeleton is directly related to its load-bearing function, which is associated with body size and mass. More than a century ago Wolff (1892) postulated that the structure of bone reflects the mechanical loading it has experienced; also, the term "functional adaptation" was proposed to refer to the process of bone remodeling resulting from its mechanical history (Roux, 1895). Later it was shown, in those with a sedentary lifestyle, that their average bone loss is greater than in more active people. Bone mass may actually be increased by weight-bearing exercise including running (Aloia et al., 1978; Dalsky et al., 1988; Eisman et al., 1991; Raab et al., 1991; Pruitt et al., 1992). However, it seems that physical exercise is not, as in children or young adults (Bassey and Ramsdale, 1994), able to increase bone mass in aging humans, in whom exercise functions to minimize bone loss (Bassey and Ramsdale, 1995; Frost, 1997).

Consideration of factors other than bone mass (such as a tendency to fall) may be important for determining which persons will have fractures, since patients with hip fractures do not appear to be more osteoporotic than a control population of the same age (Cummings, 1985). Whereas vertebral fractures seem to be caused mainly by osteoporosis alone, general frailty and inadequate motor reflexes, particularly in the elderly, are major contributing factors for hip fractures (Elffors, 1998). The latter might shift the focus of mechanisms toward neurological and psychological factors, thereby complementing the purely biomechanical models of fracture risk. Considering population shifts toward increasing longevity, projections of fracture occurrence are too conservative and the establishment of more effective risk-prevention programs becomes more important.

PHYSIOLOGY OF BONE METABOLISM

Bone is a complex tissue that serves three main purposes: it provides mechanical support for postural and locomotor activity, it is a long-term calcium reserve, and it protects hematopoietic tissue. The mineralized matrix consists of two-thirds highly ordered crystals and one-third organic component called osteoid. The mineral compartment contains 90% hydroxyapatite (Ca/P), 6% carbonate, 1% nitrate, 0.7% sodium, 0.7% magnesium, and trace elements, for example, fluoride. The osteoid component consists of 95% collagen-I which provides the framework on which bone mineral is deposited. Collagen molecules cross-link to form precisely shaped fibrils; spaces between these fibrils and the ends of collagen molecules provide initiation sites for crystal formation. Thus, calcium phosphate crystals, located predominantly between collagen fibrils, have their long axes oriented in parallel with the fibrils. Noncollagenous proteins are composed of osteonectin (23%), osteocalcin (15%), sialoprotein (9%), phosphoproteins (9%), glycoproteins (5%), proteoglycans (4%), albumin (3%), matrix Gla-protein (2%), and other proteins like decorin and biglycan. Their specific distribution and spatial relationships may be related to their function during bone resorption and formation such as recruitment, attachment, and cellular activity (Groeneveld and Burger, 2000; Ingram et al., 1993; Triffit, 1987).

The metabolic activity of bone has two objectives: it must respond to systemic needs by providing adequate calcium for use within other body compartments and, at the same time, support its own local integrity and mechanical strength. Systemic regulatory mechanisms are mainly hormonal; local mechanisms mainly, but not exclusively physicochemical (Dunston, 2000). Although these homeostatic functions are not independent—for example, an inadequate calcium supply can lead to bone demineralization, and bone disease may impair calcium balance—it is clear that the maintenance of appropriate ionized calcium content in the extracellular fluid takes precedence over maintenance of bone structural integrity.

About 5% of bone surface is covered by osteoblasts and 1% by osteoclasts. Osteoblasts arise from progenitors in connective tissue and form a continuous sheet on the surface of newly forming bone. They form collagen and other proteins, and (probably) also promote mineralization by secreting calcium-rich vesicles into the calcifying osteoid. Further, they cleave pyrophosphate by means of alkaline phosphatase, thus removing a stabilizing factor and, at the same time, increase the concentration of phosphate which promotes crystal formation. The exchange of calcium, phosphate, and other components between bone and other bodily tissues occurs across the bone membrane. The bone membrane is a continuous layer of cells comprising the periosteum, the endosteum cells that line the Haversian canals, and the osteocytes, all of which actively participate in bone mineral transport, solubilization, and crystallization. These key events are pH-dependent; they are determined by physicochemical equilibria related to the concentrations of calcium, phosphate, and other constituents in bone water; and are regulated by local mechanical peak forces as well as hormones, paracrine factors, and cytokines. Under physiologic conditions the calcium and phosphate in solution are in a metastable solution; that is, their concentration would be high enough for precipitation. However, other constituents, particularly pyrophosphate, stabilize the solution.

Both compact and trabecular bone (80% and 20% of the bone mass, respectively) have tiny chambers that contain osteocytes and interconnecting canaliculi through which osteocytes communicate by means of cytoplasmic processes. In compact bone this network provides a continuous connection between the periostal and endostal surfaces. Besides cellular components, compact bone contains extracellular (bone) fluid which forms a compartment of its own. The surface area of bone matrix that is in contact with this pool has been estimated to be 1,000 to 5,000 m^2, which is considerably more area than the entire absorptive surface within the gastrointestinal tract. Because of its sponge-like structure, trabecular bone provides more than 80% of this huge exchange interface although its mass is only about 20% of the total skeleton.

Osteocytes are the most abundant cells (10:1) of the osteoblast lineage and receive nourishment and signals by way of their gap-junction-equipped cytoplasmic processes. They are differentiated osteoblasts which became entrapped in bone matrix during growth or remodeling. Together with osteoblasts and quiescent lining cells, they compose the so-called bone membrane. The bone surface is covered mainly by flat (bone-lining) cells with few organelles, a condensed nucleus, and low metabolic activity. But they are connected to each other and to superficial osteocytes with cell processes extending into canaliculi, equipped with gap junctions, thus contributing to a syncytium formed by all bone cells except osteoclasts (Moss, 1991).

This system (Figure 7.1) comprises an information network in which each osteocyte has (probably) up to 80 cytoplasmic processes, approximately 15 mm long, arrayed in a three-dimensional manner that permits them to interconnect with up to 12 neighboring osteocytes (Palumbo et al., 1990). Neither the osteocyte nor its cytoplasmic processes entirely fills the lacuna and canaliculi in which they reside; rather, there is an extracellular space between the bone wall and cellular compartment which contains bone fluid and macromolecular complexes, with a higher proportion of large proteoglycans than in the calcified interlacunar matrix (Sauren et al., 1992). This sheath of unmineralized matrix is easily penetrated even by macromolecules. This entire arrangement provides both an intracellular (gap junctions) and an extracellular route for the rapid passage of electrical and chemical information throughout bone tissue, including osteons that are also crossed by canaliculi (Curtis et al., 1985).

The feedback mechanism by which the bone senses changes in load and initiates the deposition or resorption of bone tissue is not completely understood. Can an osteocyte or an osteoblast sense changes in the gravitational field directly and independently of changes in its environment, or does it detect those changes from its environment indirectly by contact stress? Adhesive forces on osteoblasts or osteocytes are three to four orders of magnitude larger than the gravitational forces resulting from cell weight (Cowin, 1998). Is it the magnitude or the rate of strain that is the controlling factor for local bone metabolism? Strategies for coping with the deterioration of the musculoskeletal system during long-term bed rest, immobilization, or spaceflight are dependent upon the answer to this question. It appears that the functional responses during deconditioning involve simultaneous mechanical, bioelectric, and biochemical processes.

Recent data indicate that strain affects both collagen and mineral micro-architecture, and that tensile forces are associated with increased tissue anisotropy and associated physical load (Takano et al., 1999). Bone seems to sense only time-varying forces because a constant, nontime-varying force applied to bone has the same effect as no force (Rubin and Lanyon, 1987). Thus, it would not be the absence of gravity per se that induces bone loss during spaceflight (or inactivity), but rather the time-varying force systems acting on the bone which are fundamentally altered because of ambulatory changes (Cowin, 1998).

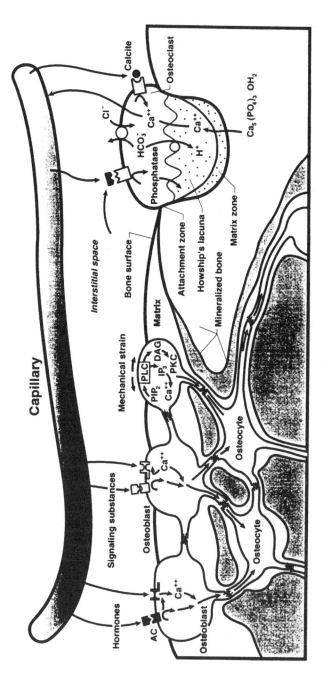

Figure 7.1 Regulation of bone formation (left) and resorption (right). Multiple plasmatic processes, equipped with gap junctions, allow osteoblasts and osteocytes cell–cell communication within the bone matrix and mineralized compacta. Osteoblasts at bone surface receive systemic (hormones) and local signaling substances by means of receptor molecules, and respond to mechanical strain. These stimuli influence calcium influx or G-protein-dependent enzyme activity (adenylate cyclase = AC, phospholipase C = PLC) and trigger second messenger mechanisms. Synthesis of organic bone substance ensues—bone gains stability where it is stressed most. Osteoclasts are activated by osteoblast-derived cytokines and prostaglandins; after forming a ring-shaped attachment zone on the surface, osteoclasts release hydrogen ions, proteases and phosphatases and form Howship's-lacunae and a matrix zone from which minerals have been dissolved. Calcium ions stimulate retraction of osteoclast processes, calcitonin reduces osteoclast motility.

It has also been suggested that fluid flow through bone interstices plays a crucial role in the transduction of extracellular mechanical phenomena to intracellular responses (Reich et al., 1990; Jones et al., 1995).

Strain-dependent propulsion of interstitial fluid through lacunar–canalicular channels contributes to the transport of nutrients, waste products, and signal molecules (Burger and Klein-Nulend, 1999), and seems to activate bone cells mechanically by means of osteoblasts or osteocytes (Turner, 1999). Osteocytes are extremely sensitive to fluid flow resulting in increased prostaglandin, as well as nitric oxide production. The osteocyte is situated to directly sense the bone strain fluid movement: peak physiological loading induces shear stresses of 0.8–3.0 Pa (Weinbaum et al., 1994) within the canaliculi, which also will strain the macromolecular connections between the osteocyte and its extracellular matrix. This transduction mechanism then would transmit information by means of integrins to the cell membrane and on to the cytoskeleton, resulting in genomic regulation within the nucleus (Wang et al., 1993; Banes et al., 1995).

Various cytokines in the osseal micro-environment regulate, at least in part, the dynamics of bone metabolism. For instance, bone represents the largest reservoir for transforming growth factor (TGF-β) which is attached to a special binding protein: TGF-β inhibits resorption by suppressing osteoclast recruitment and activity, and is a potent osteoblastic mitogen. Interleukin-6, produced by osteoblasts and stromal cells, increases bone resorption and promotes osteoclastogenesis. Some components of the insulin-like growth factor (IGF) system are also abundantly expressed in human bone: IGF-I and IGF-II are mitogens that enhance differentiation of osteoblasts. The actions of such cytokines provide a target for steroid hormones, notably estrogens and androgens (Hofbauer and Khosla, 1999).

BONE STRENGTH

Because terms such as stress, strain, strength, and elasticity are often used when discussing bone, it is important to have a clear understanding of their meaning (Cowin, 1998; Frost, 1995; Gordon, 1991):

Stress (s) is the force (f) acting in a certain direction at a certain point within a material divided by the area (A) on which the force acts; $s = f/A$. It can be expressed in any units of force over any units of area, preferably (SI standards) as $N \cdot m^{-2}$ (or Pa)[1].

Strength is usually defined as the stress that is needed to break a given material. Stress tells how *strongly* the molecules at any point in a solid material are being pulled apart. For equal strain (see below), stiffer materials generate larger stresses than more "compliant" materials. Enamel is stiffer than lamellar bone, which again is more resistant than woven bone. The ultimate "fracture force" of bone is about 130 MPa (18,855 $lb \cdot in^{-2}$). Although bone mass is highly correlated with bone strength,

---

[1]N = Newton (MN = mega-Newton, GN = giga-Newton), Pa = Pascal.

25–30% of the observed variation of bone strength is probably attributable to the cumulative and synergistic effects of other factors such as bone microstructure, architecture, and state of remodeling (Kleerekoper et al., 1985).

Strain (*e*), not to be confused with stress, tells us how *far* the molecules at any point in a solid material are being pulled apart; that is, by what proportion of the bonds between them are stretched. It is given as a relative change in length ($e = \Delta l / L$ where: l = increase of length and L = original length) and is usually expressed as a percentage. Strain is a ratio and has no units.

The *elasticity* of a given material can be characterized by the relationship between stress and strain, and is plotted in a "stress–strain diagram" the shape of which is usually not affected by the size of the tested sample. If the result is a straight line, the material is said to obey Hooke's law; the slope of the line is a measure of the material's elastic stiffness. This (constant) ratio of stress to strain is Young's elastic modulus ($E = s/e$). Obviously, E has the same dimension as stress (e.g., $MN \cdot m^{-2}$). Many common soft biological materials cannot be characterized with any standard value of E since they do not obey Hooke's law. Fresh bone has an elastic modulus of ≈ 21 $GN \cdot m^{-2}$. For comparison, human tendon has a modulus of 0.6, plywood 7.0, glass 70, and steel 210 $GN \cdot m^{-2}$.

There is disagreement concerning whether tissue anisotropy has an effect on the apparent elastic properties of cancellous bone. Using finite-element analysis with experimental data, it has been shown that the empirically observed variation of Young's moduli could be predicted to about 92% by a finite-element model (Kabel et al., 1999). Thus, an "effective isotropic tissue modulus" concept seems applicable for practical purposes.

Bone mineral density (BMD) accounts for 70–75% of bone strength (Faulkner, 2000; Heany, 1989; Ott, 1993). Several types of bone are routinely evaluated to represent the entire skeleton. The radius is used to represent the cortical bone, cancellous bone is represented by the lumbar spine, mixed bone by the proximal hip or neck of the femur, and the calcaneus is 90–95% trabecular bone. Bone density changes are used to assess altered mineralization in the lower extremities, especially during bed rest or spaceflight deconditioning. In osteoporotic persons the calcaneal mineral density is a good predictor of vertebral and femoral neck fractures (Cheng et al., 1994; Vogel et al., 1988).

Absorptiometry appears to be the most sensitive method for monitoring bone-mineral content; ultrasound techniques also provide information on bone quality (Brandenburger, 1993; Sone et al., 1998) which influences bone fragility (Schnitzler, 1993). Bone-mineral content assessment is performed using photodensitometry or photon absorptiometry and other techniques such as radiogrammetry, photon scattering, computed tomography (CT)-scan, or neutron activation analysis (Tothill, 1989); but single-photon and dual-energy absorptiometry are currently the methods of choice if BMD is the variable to be determined.

Single-photon absorptiometry is used to evaluate bones not surrounded by much soft tissue (e.g., the radius). A photon-emitting radionuclide is passed over the area to be studied, with a scintillator photon detector on the opposite side. The number of photons absorbed increases with bone density in the scanning path. The relative absorption is calibrated as bone mass (grams) per unit length of bone (centimeter). *Dual-energy absorptiometry* uses more energy so more soft tissue can be penetrated (e.g., spine, hip). Two methods are available: dual-photon absorptiometry (DPA) uses a gamma source (typically gadolinium-153 which produces 44- and 100-keV photons), whereas dual-energy x-ray absorptiometry (DEXA) works in the x-ray spectrum.

Qualitative ultrasound scanners measure the broadband ultrasound attenuation (BUA, given in decibels per megahertz; central frequency, 0.5 MHz— attenuation-based bone assessment) and the speed of sound (velocity-based bone assessment); both are referenced to the ultrasonic velocity through water at body temperature [37°C (98.6°F)]. Ultrasound interacts with bone in a fundamentally different way than electromagnetic radiation. Although high correlations can be found between bone density derived from ultrasound and electromagnetic absorption measurements (Moris et al., 1995), ultrasound propagation through bone may provide additional information on bone quality such as mechanical properties and microstructure. Therefore it is more likely to indicate the biomechanical competence of the skeleton (Kaufman and Einhorn, 1993). BUA can identify hip fractures with an 80% sensitivity (Baran et al., 1988) and is now widely used in both clinical and experimental settings, including spaceflight medical investigations.

Quantitative computed tomography (QCT) of vertebral bones produces high errors (10–30%) because of variations in marrow fat and osteoid (Mazess and Whedon, 1983): it can be used as a valid indicator of neither vertebral strength nor whole-body bone density. QCT could predict femoral and hip fracture risk, but the radiation dose is much higher than that of DPA. For these reasons QCT is not recommended for BMD assessment.

Early intervention in patients with osteopenia is necessary to prevent its progression to osteoporosis. Bone density should generally exceed 1 $g \cdot cm^{-2}$, and it is reported as a standard deviation from mean values: osteopenia is defined as 1.0–2.5 SD below normal; and osteoporosis as >2.5 SD below normal. Osteoporosis is indicated by a >10% density loss relative to a reference value matched for sex, age, height, weight, and race. Density values between 0.80 and 0.99 $g \cdot cm^{-2}$ are associated with less than a 20% chance of spontaneous fractures, whereas values <0.62 g/cm^2 are indicative of a twofold increase in fracture risk.

BIOCHEMICAL MARKERS OF BONE METABOLISM

Bone is in a dynamic state—being broken down continuously (resorption) and reformed (formation) by the action of osteoblasts and osteoclasts, respectively. Bone metabolism occurs at the bone surface at focused sites termed bone metabolism units (BMUs). At any given time there are about 1 million BMUs in various phases of the bone cycle; as much as 25% of trabecular bone and 3% of cortical bone is resorbed and replaced each year (Parfitt, 1994).

Both resorption and formation give rise to the release of several "markers" into the bloodstream. Consequently, concentration changes of these markers are used to assess the dynamic state of bone, but none provides unambiguous information on the skeleton's actual remodeling balance; however, local gain of bone mass in one location along with bone loss in another probably blurs the picture.

If activation is initiated on a particular bone site, osteoclasts are attracted to the new BMU where they erode the matrix to form a dip (Howship's lacuna, Figure 7.1). Each osteoclast forms a tight sealing zone at the "outer rim" of the developing lacuna and releases numerous lysosomal and nonlysosomal substances such as lysozyme, phosphatase, glucuronidase, collagenases, and hydrogen ions. It takes approximately 1 week for the lacuna to reach a depth of about 50 μm at which time resorption stops, the osteoclast detaches, and osteoblasts are recruited to the BMU. They lay down new osteoid into the lacuna, beginning at its bottom and proceeding until the hole is again filled giving the site increased tensile strength. The entire process takes up to 80 days; however, mineralization of the newly formed matrix is initiated soon by also moving bottom-up in parallel with osteoid formation. The remodeled area finally passes into a quiescent phase to complete the bone cycle which takes 2–3 months. Incomplete filling by osteoblasts (as in older men) or exaggerated erosion by osteo-clasts (as in postmenopausal women) create a deficit in osseous mechanical strength and, therefore, fracture risk.

Assessment of bone turnover should be based on those sequences of bone cycle. Resorption markers should reflect osteoclast activity or collagen degradation; formation markers, on the other hand, should reflect osteoblastic synthetic activity or extracellular metabolism of procollagen. The "markers" described below are utilized (Blumsohn and Eastell, 1997; Calvo et al., 1996; Christenson, 1997; Epstein, 1988; Garnero and Delmas, 1998).

Resorption Markers

Urinary calcium

Fasting urine calcium concentration lacks diagnostic value because it is affected by variations in diet, metabolism, renal function, and hormone activity levels. Nonetheless, calcium excretion has been frequently monitored in astronauts and bed-rested subjects to assess general bone mineral loss. Urinary calcium loss occurs during the entire duration of bed rest (Greenleaf and Kozlowski, 1982; Krasnoff and Painter, 1999).

Acid phosphatase

Five acid phosphatase (AP) isoenzymes have been identified; their major sources are bone, prostatic gland, platelets, red cells, and the spleen. Osteoclasts produce high amounts of the bone isoenzyme which "leaks" into the bloodstream during resorption and after detachment of the osteoclast's sealing zone. Bone AP retains its activity after treatment with L(+)tartrate, so tartrate-resistant acid phosphatase (TRAP) is indicative of the level of bone isoenzyme, although this measure is not entirely specific. A monoclonal immunoassay for bone AP has been developed, but it also lacks specificity. Serum has higher AP activity than plasma because erythrocytes release AP during the *in-vitro* clotting process; and AP is unstable without special treatment to lower its pH. Thus, it can be concluded that characterization of AP as a marker of bone metabolism is incomplete. Consequently, its use in spaceflight or bed rest studies is limited.

Hydroxyproline

Post-translational hydroxylation of collagen-residue prolin gives rise to hydroxyproline (HP) which comprises about 13% of collagen. After collagen breakdown HP is not reutilized; instead it is catabolized (90%) or excreted as small peptides by the kidneys. Consequently, urine HP can be used as a marker of bone breakdown. However, one procollagen extension peptide (PINP, see below) which emerges during bone formation also gives rise to HP excretion. Furthermore, inflammation also elevates urinary HP level because the complement factor C1q contains a sequence similar to that of collagen. Finally, HP is present in the diet, particularly in gelatine-containing food (urine sampling after an overnight fast eliminated dietary effects on HP excretion). In summary, HP excretion is a suitable bone resorption marker if potential errors can be excluded, and HP excretion has often been employed as an indicator of bone loss in spaceflight and bed rest studies (Ellis, Welch, and Prescott, 1979; Lockwood et al., 1979; Schneider, 1991; Smith et al., 1977; Van der Weil, 1991).

Galactosyl hydroxylysine

Hydroxylysine is a modified amino acid peculiar to collagens. Its glycosylated form, galactosyl hydroxylysine (GHyl), is probably not reused after collagen degradation and it is not absorbed in significant amounts from the diet. Because of tissue-specific differences in the ratios of GHyl, and its glucosylated form (Glc.GHyl) which mostly emanates from skin collagens, GHyl is relatively specific to bone degradation (Pinnell et al., 1971; Krane et al., 1977). In urine, 80% of the total hydroxylysine appears as glycoside, 10% is free, and 10% is peptide-bound; this 80/20 ratio is age-dependent because the free and peptide-bound fractions are most prominent in the urine of infants and children (Askenasi, 1975). GHyl has been used as an indicator of bone collagen destruction in recent deconditioning investigations (Al-Dehaimi et al., 1999).

Telopeptides

During resorption the osteoclasts degrade collagen to small fractions [N-telopeptides (NTX) and C-telopeptides (CTX)] which are specific for bone resorption since different fractions are formed during breakdown of nonskeletal collagen. They are released into the circulation and readily pass through renal glomeruli into the urine. Although several factors can interfere with renal elimination of NTX and CTX, their excretion is fairly specific for bone degradation. Serum type I collagen cross-linked

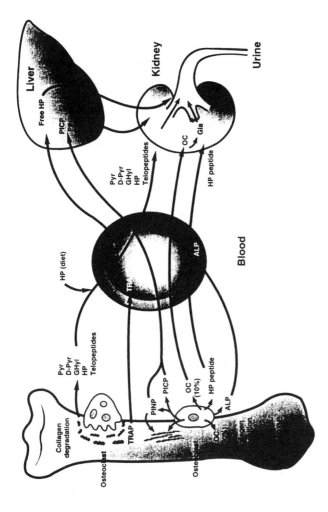

Figure 7.2 Bone biomarkers are transported by the bloodstream, to be partly degraded by the liver and partly excreted by the kidneys. *Resorption markers*: Cleavage of bone collagen produces several compounds: hydroxyproline (HP), galactosyl hydroxylysine (GHyl), hydroxypyridinium cross-links (Pyr and DPyr), C- and N-telopeptides. Much of the free HP is reabsorbed in the kidneys and oxidized in the liver; dietary HP may enter the circulation and increase total blood level. Circulating products containing cross-links largely vary in magnitude (few amino acids to large telopeptides). TRAP = tartrate-resistant acid phosphatase. *Formation markers*: After having been "clipped" from procollagen-I, the carboxy- and amino-terminal peptide ends PINP and PICP are mostly released to the bloodstream and are degraded by the liver. Osteocalcin (OC) to a large part enters the matrix after having been formed, a small fraction escapes to the blood; renal catabolism liberates free carboxyglutamic acid (Gla) and Gla-peptides into the urine. Bone alkaline phosphatase (ALP) derives from active osteoblasts.

C-telopeptide (ICTP) seems to be a reliable bone resorption marker (Eriksen et al., 1993) and has been used in bed rest investigations (Zerwekh et al., 1998).

Pyridinoline cross-links

Stabilization of mature collagen and elastin requires the formation of pyridinoline (Pyr) and deoxypyridinoline (D-Pyr) cross-links (Figure 7.2). These are formed by post-translational processing of lysine and hydroxylysine, mainly in bone tissue, and are released into the extracellular fluid after bone degradation without being metabolized. This makes them fairly specific resorption markers; 60% are bound to plasma protein and the remaining 40% are filtered and excreted in the urine (Kamel et al., 1995). Pyr and D-Pyr are widely used in investigations of deconditioning (Nishimura et al., 1994; Smith et al., 1998), and D-Pyr is found almost exclusively in bone (Eyre et al., 1984). Pyr and D-Pyr excretion has been determined during long-term spaceflight (Smith et al., 1999).

Formation Markers

Procollagen-I extension peptides

Procollagen-I is an osteoblast-derived precursor of collagen. Its carboxy- and amino-terminal peptide ends are "clipped" during post-translational extracellular processing giving rise to the carboxyterminal propeptide (PICP) and aminoterminal peptide (PINP) of procollagen-I. The PICP is taken up by mannose receptors and PINP by scavenger receptors of endothelial cells in the liver. Hepatic clearance must be considered when quantifying serum PICP and PINP levels, which should be good markers of bone formation. PIPC reflects the first step of osteoblastic differentiation because it is linked to collagen synthesis (Risteli and Risteli, 1993).

Alkaline phosphatase

The second step of osteoblastic differentiation—enabling matrix maturation—releases alkaline phosphatase (ALP) into the systemic circulation. Blood carries four isoenzymes that are somewhat specific for liver, bone, intestines, and placenta. The tetrameric bone-specific isoenzyme (B-ALP, a glycoprotein) is produced by osteo-blasts and is involved in bone mineralization, probably by means of a breakdown of pyrophosphate which inhibits calcium phosphate deposition. The B-ALP, an excellent indicator of general bone formation, is released into the circulation in dimeric form after cleavage by a phospholipase (Howard et al., 1987). Numerous assays are available for serum B-ALP measurement.

Osteocalcin

Mature osteoblasts produce osteocalcin (OC) (or BGP for bone gla protein), a vitamin-K-dependent calcium-binding peptide which is one of the bone matrix's most abundant noncollagenous proteins. Being connected to matrix mineralization, it represents the final step of osteoblastic differentiation (Risteli and Risteli, 1993). Osteocalcin is mainly deposited in the bone matrix during formation, whereas about 15% of it escapes into the circulation where it can be detected in both intact and fragmented forms (Delmas et al., 1985). When bone is resorbed some of the deposited OC is degraded, but up to 70% enters the circulation. Therefore, plasma OC may be both newly synthesized during formation and released during resorption. When the two processes are uncoupled, OC is considered a marker of osteoblast activity; otherwise its serum level mirrors the paramount intensity of bone turnover.

RESULTS FROM BED REST STUDIES

Removal of mechanical loading leads to muscle atrophy as well as to increased bone resorption such as that observed with disuse during body casting (Deitrick et al., 1948; Patel et al., 1969; Sargeant et al., 1977) or prolonged bed rest (BR) without exercise training (Krupina et al., 1982; Saltin et al., 1968). The similarities in calcium and bone changes during long-term spaceflight and BR-deconditioning are striking: decreased bone formation, increased bone resorption, continued urinary and fecal calcium loss, bone redistribution, decreased plasma $1,25(OH)_2D$ (the biologically active form of vitamin D), and no consistent changes in plasma parathyroid hormone (Bikle et al., 1997; Bloomfield, 1997; Zerwekh et al., 1998). Bone mineral losses during prolonged deconditioning may well exceed 10% per year (LeBlanc et al., 1990). Urinary and fecal calcium excretion are increased by 20–50% (Arnaud et al., 1992; Van der Weil et al., 1991; Zerwekh et al., 1998). Calcium loss begins a few days into BR and stays elevated, leading to ever-increasing negative calcium balance (Greenleaf and Kozlowski, 1982; Krasnoff and Painter, 1999).

During 4 months of BR-deconditioning average bone mineral density decreases by about 1% per month in the spine, pelvis, and femur, together with increased osteoclastic activity (biopsy) and decreased mineralization parameters; pyridinoline cross-link excretion was elevated and calcium absorption and $1,25(OH)_2D$ levels were decreased. More than 10% of the bone mass was lost from the calcanei and 3% from femoral neck and spine, but skull bone density increased by 3% (Chappard et al., 1989; LeBlanc et al., 1990, 1995; Vico et al., 1987). Thus, the BR data are consistent with spaceflight results in that bones that encounter the largest gravitational stress with ambulation in a 1-G environment experience the greatest losses in bone mineral content when this mechanical load is removed. The loss of calcaneal mass reflects the marked decrease of force normally exerted by muscles inserting onto the Achilles' tendon during standing, walking, and running. The associated antigravity muscles, such as the triceps surae, also undergo the greatest atrophy during weightlessness and BR (Grigoryeva and Kozlovskaya, 1987).

The upper extremities maintain or even increase their bone density, probably because the workload on the arms is maintained or even elevated during deconditioning. The cause for increased bone mass in the skull is not clear; it might be a result of increased hydrostatic forces in the upper body caused by the cephalad fluid

	wk 1-2	wk 3-4	wk 5-8	wk 9-12	4 mo	6 mo
≈+200%						ICTP DPyr
+60-120%					ICTP	Pyr
+40-60%		NTX	HP NTX	DPyr HP ICTP NTX Pyr	DPyr tr. re. s.	
+20-40%	HP NTX uCa	DPyr HP ICTP Pyr uCa	DPyr ICTP Pyr uCa	uCa		
≈+10%	P Pyr	P	P	P		
≈+2%	sCa	sCa	sCa	sCa		
-2–4%						Tib/fem/sp
≈-10%						Calc
-15–40%	1,25D	1,25D PTH	1,25D PTH	1,25D PTH		
≈-50%					e. os. s.	

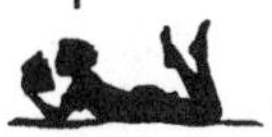

Figure 7.3 Time-course of changes during bed rest deconditioning. Inset: Incorrect posture—maximum head inclination 30°, legs must not be elevated above horizontal. calc = bone mineral density in calcaneus; DPyr = urinary deoxypyridinoline cross-link excretion; e. os. s. = extent of osteoid surface; HP = urinary hydroxyproline excretion; ICTP = serum type I C-telopeptide concentration; NTX = urinary N-telopeptide excretion; P = serum phosphate concentration and urinary phosphate excretion; PTH = serum parathormone concentration; Pyr = urinary pyridinoline cross-link excretion; sCa = serum calcium concentration; tr. re. s. = trabecular resorption surface; uCa = urinary calcium excretion; tib / fem/ sp = bone mineral density in tibia, femur, and spine; 1,25D = serum vitamin D [1,25(OH)$_2$D] concentration. (From Arnaud et al., 1992; Fiore et al., 1998; Leblanc et al., 1990; Palle et al., 1992; Smith et al., 1998; Van der Weil et al., 1991; Vico et al., 1987; Zerwekh et al., 1998.).

shifts that occur both in weightlessness and during horizontal and head-down body positioning (Bikle et al., 1997).

Overall, bone loss saturates urinary calcium excretion despite gradually decreasing intestinal calcium absorption—from 31 to 24% of dietary intake over 17 weeks of horizontal BR (LeBlanc et al., 1995)—causing hypercalciuria and highly increased risk of kidney stone formation (Sawin, 1998). Increased fecal calcium loss eventually accounts for 50% of the negative calcium balance observed after 2 months of BR. Bone biopsies in 20 healthy males after 4 months of BR showed an increase of about 50% in bone resorption surface (Bloomfield, 1997; Vico et al., 1987). The Pyr cross-link excretion increased, but parathormone, calcitonin, osteocalcin, and B-ALP plasma levels were not altered significantly (LeBlanc et al., 1995; Smith et al., 1998; Zerwekh et al., 1998). However, in patients with functionally complete immobilization where muscular activity has ceased, consistently low parathormone levels have been observed (Bergmann et al., 1977).

In 50 male and female stroke-immobilized (30–180 days) patients aged 47–74 yr, bone resorption markers increased continually with deconditioning duration (urinary Pyr and D-Pyr excretion reached doubled to tripled values after 6 months BR, as did serum ICTP concentration), whereas formation markers (B-ALP, PIPC) remained within the normal range in all patients regardless of the duration of the immobilization (Fiore et al., 1998). Thus, it seems that during BR immobilization an uncoupling occurs between bone formation and resorption such that bone collagen breakdown is not a self-limiting process, but is ongoing.

Biphosphonate treatment, together with a 1–2 hr/day exercise program, proved effective in reducing BR-induced bone loss (Chappard et al., 1989; Grigoriev et al., 1992). The time course of changes of biochemical markers for osseal metabolism seems to indicate that antiresorptive drugs might serve as a useful countermeasure for deconditioning-induced bone loss (Zerwekh et al., 1998). However, it remains an open question as to what extent physical exertion and antiresorptive therapy, singly or combined, can substitute for the loss of mechanical loading resulting from postural control, locomotion, and upright exercise in a weightless or BR environment.

In summary, results from long-duration BR studies in healthy persons without application of countermeasures indicate that bone loss is similar to, or possibly lower than, that measured during spaceflight (Figure 7.3). The biochemical changes that precede bone loss occur quite rapidly: according to marker time-profiles, bone resorption is elevated as early as the first days of deconditioning (Van der Weil et al., 1991; Smith et al., 1998). About 0.2 g of calcium per day is lost; calcium absorption is decreased; bone resorption markers are elevated, seemingly rising continually with duration of deconditioning; formation markers remain unaltered; and plasma $1,25(OH_2)$-D is decreased. Bone biopsies revealed increased osteoclastic activity and reduced bone formation and mineralization (Vico et al., 1987).

Because of ethical considerations, the effects of very long-duration immobilization may never be studied. However, there is one documented extreme "case study." A young man went to bed in 1932 and remained there for the rest of his life. After 50 years of "bed rest," his limbs were "thin as the legs of a ladder-back chair" (Fortney et al., 1996). This observation supports the hypothesis that with reduced hydrostatic pressure and inadequate mechanical stimulation, muscle and bone losses continue until no more tissue is left to be absorbed.

RESULTS FROM SPACEFLIGHT

Extended-duration spaceflight provides another mode for studying the effects of low mechanical stimulation and accompanying bone loss over long time periods in otherwise fit and healthy humans. Changes in astronauts' bone structure that occur with weightlessness deconditioning do not constitute true systemic osteoporosis: only weight-bearing bones of the lower body extremities lose mass, whereas those in the upper body remain more or less unaffected or even gain substance. A large percentage of bone fractures on Earth in ambulatory people occur in the hip region, and the overall adaptation—including metabolic alterations and endocrine responses—to reduced physical loading seems to be very similar in the various models of deconditioning with bone loss.

The question whether exposure to weightlessness per se can influence bone cell metabolism (Burger and Klein-Mulend, 1998), or if reduced mechanical loading of the skeleton functions by means of systemic–structural effects at the interface of the cellular environment, seems to be resolved. Induced bone loss in humans as a result of direct gravitation sensing by the osteocytes or osteoblasts is highly unlikely because constant, nonvarying force applied to bone has the same effect as no force (Rubin and Lanyon, 1987). Thus, a change in effective gravity, as with BR-deconditioning or spaceflight, has essentially no effect on the single bone cell but a major effect on the intact skeleton. Bone cells receive information on changes in the gravity field from their contact environment; a 1-G stress on an isolated cell is too weak to be perceived (Cowin, 1998). However, several days of weightlessness can reduce the differentiation of osteoblastic cells in response to growth-promoting signal substances (Carmeliet et al., 1998).

One of the first studies of bone loss from human spaceflight emerged from the Gemini program; there was reduction in bone density with mineral loss in the os calcis of 2.9–9.2% after 4–14 days of weightlessness (Mack et al., 1967; Vose, 1974). Further, metabolic studies revealed increased urinary calcium and phosphate excretion in the Gemini VII astronauts (Lutwak et al., 1969). Later, Apollo 17 astronauts exhibited a small but significant loss of total body weight, a 0.2% loss of total body calcium, and a 0.7% loss of total body phosphorus after this 14-day flight; mainly a result of increased fecal (calcium, phosphorus) and urinary (calcium) excretion (Rambaut et al., 1975).

These mass and mineral losses were comparable to those reported in BR studies of similar duration, and were confirmed in other studies that indicated increased calcium excretion as well (Johnson et al., 1973; Lutwak et al., 1969) including data from the 28-day Skylab II mission, where calcium loss was about 120 mg/day with increased phosphorus and nitrogen excretion (Whedon et al., 1975) plus decreased mineral content, especially in the os calcis and radius (Vogel and Whittle, 1976b). Reduced bone mineral content was also reported in Apollo crews (Vogel and Whittle, 1976a). Later, bone-related hormones were measured in Spacelab shuttle astronauts and only transient increases in $1,25(OH)_2D$ levels were found; all other parameters remained unchanged (Morey-Holton et al., 1988). During a 115-day spaceflight, urinary Pyr and D-Pyr excretion was increased and in three subjects plasma B-ALP was diminished (Smith et al., 1999). Surprisingly, after 8 months in orbit, MIR space station occupants had no clear evidence of altered vertebral bone mineral density (Oganov et al., 1991), whereas reduced bone mineral density in the pelvis and femoral neck and trochanter occurred in others after up to 10 months of flight (Schneider et al., 1992). Preflight and postflight measurements accompanying

8-month missions revealed, in contrast to the hypothesized loss of trabecular bone from the vertebral body because of unloading, that there was little or no bone loss at this site—a finding that apparently validates the effectiveness of the exercise training regimen for preventing spinal bone loss, as well as minimizing calcaneal losses (Oganov et al., 1990).

The Russian inflight exercise countermeasure program for cosmonauts induced the vertical loads produced on the bones during normal ambulation or running on Earth, but it did not exercise the antigravity postural muscles in the back. These muscles hold the body erect while standing or help return the torso to its normal position when twisting movements are performed. Mechanical load exerted by these muscles on the spine are not transmitted to the vertebral bodies, but to the transverse and spinous bony processes to which the muscles are attached; consequently, if those muscles are not exercised they will not load the bone. Analysis of CT data showed that even though the vertebral bodies did not lose bone, the posterior elements lost 8% which accompanied a 4% decrease in the volume of the muscles attached to the bone (Oganov et al., 1990).

Because most space missions do not last longer than 6 months, there are inadequate data for use in estimating the ultimate extent of bone loss after longer flights. After 1 year in orbit one cosmonaut lost 10% of his trabecular bone from the upper lumbar vertebrae, and another gained 5% mineral density (Grigoriev et al., 1991). However, for two cosmonauts in space for more than 300 days, the rate of bone loss in their spine was about half the overall body average, whereas changes in their lower legs were average (LeBlanc et al., 1998). These findings suggest that bone loss continues only where the mechanical stimulation remains very low despite the bungee cord, treadmill, and cycle exercises performed in orbit; whereas the rate of loss decreases in other skeletal regions.

Although stress-related hormones (e.g., plasma levels of cortisol and IGF-1) remained unresponsive, extended-duration spaceflight resulted in not only strongly depressed bone formation, but also increased bone resorption (Caillot-Augusseau et al., 1998); others, however have failed to find evidence of increased resorption activity (Collet et al., 1997). This discrepancy probably reflects different mission profiles and circumstances which also occur in BR investigations (LeBlanc et al., 1990). A consistent finding is low in-flight and increased post-flight plasma PTH levels which can be explained as a consequence of changed bone remodeling; that is, calcium loss in-flight and hyper-remodeling after landing (Caillot-Augusseau et al., 1998; LeBlanc et al., 1998). Short-term changes inflight seem to occur only in trabecular bone of the lower legs (weight-bearing bones); whereas after several months in orbit a more general disuse degradation ensues, comparable to the generalized bone loss observed in the iliac crest of paraplegic patients (Collet et al., 1997). When bone loss is regional; that is, when it is limited primarily to the weight-bearing bones, the whole-body change in biochemical markers provides even more convincing evidence for the role of bone resorption because the response must be even greater if it is from a smaller portion of the skeleton. International standardization of experimental protocols will increase the significance of results (Miyamoto et al., 1998).

BONE RECOVERY AFTER DECONDITIONING

It has been proposed that recovery of lost bone requires a longer period of time than the duration of the deconditioning (Smith et al., 1977; Collet et al., 1997). Although serum calcium concentration (which is particularly fine-tuned by endocrine regulation) returns to control values immediately after reambulation, serum phosphate concentration as well as urinary calcium excretion may still be elevated for 1 week after an equal duration of BR; reduced $1,25(OH)_2D$ levels also have been observed as serum PTH and urinary phosphate excretion are back to control values at this point (Arnaud et al., 1992; Van der Wiel et al., 1991; Zerwekh et al., 1998). After 6 weeks $1,25(OH)_2D$ serum levels are restored, but resorption markers (e.g., hydroxyproline excretion) remain elevated, while serum phosphate levels are decreased at this point in a study where complete immobilization including muscle relaxant drug application was applied on 14 patients with lumbar disc protrusion (Van der Wiel et al., 1991). Thus, after short-term deconditioning, significant alterations may be found even 6 weeks after reambulation.

With regard to spaceflight: 4–12 weeks in orbit produced partly significant post-landing urinary resorption marker excretion (N-telopeptides, Pyr, and D-Pyr cross-links) for up to 3 weeks in the Skylab 2 crew (4 weeks in orbit), the Skylab 3 crew (9 weeks in orbit), and the Skylab 4 crew (12 weeks in orbit). Data from this investigation were the first to demonstrate that bone resorption is elevated during spaceflight (Smith et al., 1998).

Twelve days of reambulation after a 12-week period of strict horizontal BR (no head elevation exceeding 30°, only horizontal limb movements allowed) failed to bring back resorption markers (urinary hydroxyproline and D-Pyr excretion) in 11 subjects who also displayed increased serum PICP and decreased $1,25(OH)_2D$ and calcium levels (Zerwekh et al., 1998). In another study, up to 7 weeks after finishing a 17-week horizontal BR period in eight male subjects, urinary excretion of resorption markers seemingly remained above pre-BR control (but $p > 0.05$ because of large individual differences) (Smith et al., 1998).

LeBlanc et al. (1990) quantified bone loss and recovery from long-term disuse (17 weeks of strict horizontal BR) in six male volunteers by monitoring bone mineral density (BMD) from total-body scans at the lumbar spine, hip, tibia, forearm, calcaneus, and segmental regions. The time-course of BMD was estimated by linear regression, using data points derived from the sampling sites both during and after deconditioning. Whereas a 1% increase in BMD in the radius and a 2% decrease in the tibia were completely reversed after 6 months of reambulation, the ≈4% BMD reduction at the lumbar spine and femoral neck remained unchanged after 6 months of reambulation. A more than 10% BMD reduction ensued at the calcaneus with 4-months of BR; after 6 months of reambulation the remaining loss was <2%.

When do physicians need to start worrying about bone loss in BR patients? Not after a few days, but things get worse with increasing duration of deconditioning: excess calcium excretion brings risk of kidney stone formation; material loss from weight-bearing bones like the calcaneus may exceed 3% per month; losses from the spine and femur might be irreversible; and, last but not least, the rate of bone loss increases in the presence of additional stress factors that are typical for a clinical setting.

Whereas the hip and spine lose an average of 1% bone mineral per month of BR or spaceflight in healthy people (double this figure in individual cases; LeBlanc et al., 1990), comparison of these results with those of clinical studies of injured patients reveals that the rate of bone loss may be much greater than reported for deconditioning alone: 4–8 times in the spine (Hansson et al., 1975; Krolner and Toft, 1983; Mazess and Whedon, 1983), and 6–12 times in the tibia following non-fracture injury (Andersson and Nilsson, 1979). Thus, injury and general catabolic state increase the rate of bone loss during physiologic adaptation to deconditioning by up to one order of magnitude. Countermeasures like exercise should be applied early, and they need to be targeted primarily at the spine and hip.

OUTLOOK

There are still unanswered questions about the extent to which the bone lost during deconditioning is unavoidable. Investigations into the physiology of counter-measures applied separately or combined under clearly defined conditions, and using state-of-the-art methods, will continue to provide valuable data that will help to increase our understanding of bone physiology (Skerry, 1997). Studies of this kind almost always produce important spinoffs for health protection, diagnostics, and therapeutic measures, not only because the data can be applied to everyday medical use, but also because they challenge the functional paradigms we take for granted. Weightlessness, combined with the unavoidable isolation (and potentially perfect monitoring) of spacefaring humans, still provides a unique and extremely important research opportunity.

LeBlanc et al. (1998) have suggested a number of factors that should be considered in deconditioning-related bone research:

1. Current data suggest that several years may be required for complete recovery of bone lost after extended-duration spaceflight; the degree and rate of this reversal of bone loss is not adequately known.

2. How much is the fracture risk increased after long-term bed rest or space-flight deconditioning? This information would allow rational assessment of how much protection is needed after certain periods of bone loss from disuse.

3. None of the presently used countermeasures has yet been proved completely effective; others are needed.

4. More data on bone remodeling are needed, particularly monitoring of bio-chemical markers combined with physical measurements.

5. Intestinal absorption at different points in time should be quantitated further using stable tracers.

6. More data are needed on local distribution of bone loss (which may be quite inhomogeneous in a given bone), especially sub-regional measurements of bone architecture.

7. Physiological conditions such as general stress, nutrition, fluid shifts, dehydration, and bone prefusion should be emphasized.

8. The ability to better predict the amount of bone loss expected under certain circumstances should be refined.

Bone has fascinating features because it is a living, adaptive, dynamic tissue that presents a multitude of research aspects—physical, biomolecular, cellular (signal processing, extracellular adhesion mechanisms), endocrine, systemic, and clinical. Have those challenges received adequate attention from the scientific community? Does the discipline of skeletal physiology suffer from "poor interdisciplinary communication" (Frost, 1997)? If so, the problem would be by no means unique, but rather typical in our era of specialized, speed-driven, reductionistic research. Bone loss resulting from conditions like microgravity or from prolonged BR-deconditioning, and increased skeletal stress with hypergravity or vibration, constitute complex problems; ones that require transdisciplinary, integrative, biological, and medical investigation.

REFERENCES

Al-Dehaimi, A. W., Blumsohn, A., and Eastell, R. (1999) Serum galactosyl hydroxylysine as a biochemical marker of bone resorption. *Clin. Chem.* **45**: 676–681.

Aloia, J. F., Cohn, S. H., Babu, T., Abesamis, C., Kalici, N., and Ellis, K. (1978) Skeletal mass and body composition in marathon runners. *Metabolism* **27**: 1793–1796.

Andersson, S. M., and Nilsson, B. E. (1979) Changes in bone mineral content following ligamentous knee injuries. *Med. Sci. Sports* **11**: 351–353.

Arnaud, S. B., Sherrard, D. J., Maloney, N., Whalen, R. T., and Fung, P. (1992) Effects of 1-week head-down tilt bed rest on bone formation and the calcium endocrine system. *Aviat. Space Environ. Med.* **63**: 14–20.

Askenasi, R. (1975) Urinary excretion of free hydroxylysine, peptide-bound hydroxylysine and hydroxylysyl glycosides in physiological conditions. *Clin. Chim. Acta* **59**: 87–92.

Banes, A. J., Tsuzaki, M., Yamamoto, J., Fischer, T., Brigman, B., Brown, T., and Miller, L. (1995) Mechanoreception at the cellular level: the detection, interpretation, and diversity of responses to mechanical signals. *Biochem. Cell. Biol.* **73**: 349–365.

Baran, D. T., Kelly, A. M., Kerellas, A., Gionet, M., Proce, M., Leahey, D., Steuterman, S., McSherry, B., and Roche, J. (1988) Ultrasound attenuation of the calcaneus in women with osteoporosis and hip fractures. *Calcif. Tissue Int.* **43**: 138–142.

Bassey, E. J., and Ramsdale, S. J. (1994) Increase in femoral bone density in young women following high-impact exercise. *Osteoporos. Int.* **4**: 72–75.

Bassey, E. J., and Ramsdale, S. J. (1995) Weight-bearing exercise and ground reaction forces: a 12-month randomized controlled trial of effects on bone-mineral density in healthy postmenopausal women. *Bone* **16**: 469–476.

Bergmann, P. A., Heilporn, A., Schoutens, A., Paternot, J., and Tricot, A. (1977) Longitudinal study of calcium and bone metabolism in paraplegic patients. *Paraplegia* **15**: 147–159.

Bikle, D. D., Halloran, B. P., and Morey-Holton, E. (1997) Space flight and the skeleton: lessons for the earthbound. *Endocrinologist* **7**: 10–22.

Bloomfield, S. A. (1997) Changes in musculoskeletal structure and function with prolonged bed rest. *Med. Sci. Sports Exerc.* **29**: 197–206.

Blumsohn, A., and Eastell, R. (1997) The performance and utility of biochemical markers of bone turnover: do we know enough to use them in clinical practice? *Ann. Clin. Biochem.* **34**: 449–459.

Boissy, P., Machuca, I., Pfaff, M., Ficheux, D., and Jurdic, P. (1998) Aggregation of mononucleated precursors triggers cell surface expression of alpha v beta 3 integrin, essential to formation of osteoclast-like multinucleated cells. *J. Cell Sci.* **111**: 2563–2574.

Brandenburger, G. H. (1993) Clinical determination of bone quality: is ultrasound the answer? *Calcif. Tissue Int.* **53**: S151–S156.

Burger, E. H., and Klein-Nulend, J. (1998) Microgravity and bone cell mechanosensitivity. *Bone* **22**: 127S-30.

Burger, E. H., and Klein-Nulend, J. (1999) Mechanotransduction in bone: role of the lacuno-canalicular network. *FASEB J.* **13**: S101–S112.

Caillot-Augusseau, A., Lafage-Proust, M. H., Soler, C., Pernod, J., Dubois, F., and Alexandre, C.(1998) Bone formation and resorption biological markers in cosmonauts during and after a 180-day space flight (Euromir 95). *Clin. Chem.* **44**: 578–585.

Calvo, M. S., Eyre, D. R., and Gundberg, C. M.(1996) Molecular basis and clinical application of biological markers of bone turnover. *Endocr. Rev.* **17**: 333–368.

Carmeliet, G., Nys, G., Stockmans, I., and Bouillon, R. (1998) Gene expression related to the differentiation of osteoblastic cells is altered by microgravity. *Bone* **22**: 139S–143S.

Chappard, D., Alexandre, C., Palle, S., Vico, L., and Morukov, B. V. (1989) Effects of a biphosphonate on osteoclast number during prolonged bed rest in healthy humans. *Metabolism* **38**: 822–825.

Cheng, S., Suominen, H., Era, P., and Heikkinen, E. (1994) Bone density of the calcaneus and fractures in 75- and 80-year old men and women. *Osteoporos. Int.* **4**: 48–54.

Christenson, R. H. (1997) Biochemical markers of bone metabolism: an overview. *Clin. Biochem.* **30**: 573–93.

Collet, P., Uebelhart, D., Vico, L., Moro, L., Hartmann, D., Roth, M., and Alexandre, C. (1997) Effects of 1- and 6-month spaceflight on bone mass and biochemistry in two humans. *Bone* **20**: 547–551.

Cowin, S. C. (1998) On mechanosensation in bone under microgravity. *Bone* **22**: S119–S125.

Cummings, S. R. (1985) Are patients with hip fractures more osteoporotic? *Am. J. Med.* **78**: 487–494.

Curtis, T. A., Ashrafi, S. H., and Weber, D. F. (1985) Canalicular communication in the cortices of human long bones. *Anat. Rec.* **212**: 336–344.

Dalsky, G. P., Stocke, K. S., Ehsani, A. A., Lee, W. C., and Birge, S. J. (1988) Weightbearing exercise training and lumbar bone mineral content in postmenopausal women. *Ann. Intern. Med.* **108**: 824–828.

Deitrick, J. E., Whedon, G. D., Shorr, E., Toscani, V., and Davis, V. B. (1948) Effect of immobilization on metabolic and physiologic functions of normal men. *Am. J. Med.* **4**: 3–35.

Delmas, P. D., Malaval, L., Arlot, M. E., and Meunier, P. L. (1985) Serum bone GLA-protein compared to bone histomorphometry in endocrine diseases. *Bone* **6**: 339–341.

Dunston, C. R. (2000) Osteoprotegerin and osteoprotegerin ligand mediate the local regulation of bone resorption. *Endocrinology* **10**: 18–26.

Eisman, J. A., Sambrook, P. N., Kelly, P. J., and Pocock, N. A. (1991) Exercise and its interaction with genetic influences in the determination of bone mineral density. *Am. J. Med.* **91**: (S5B): 5–9.

Elffors, L. (1998) Are osteoporotic fractures due to osteoporosis? Impacts of a frailty pandemic in an aging world. *Aging Clin. Exp. Res.* **10**: 191–204.

Ellis, J. P., Jr., Welch, B. E., and Prescott, J. M. (1972) Effects of hypercapernia and physical deconditioning on musculoskeletal protein in man. *Aerospace Med.* **43**: 22–27.

Epstein, S. (1988) Serum and urinary markers of bone remodeling: assessment of bone turnover. *Endocr. Rev.* **9**: 437–449.

Eriksen, E. F., Charles, P., Melsen, F., Mosekilde, L., Risteli, L., and Risteli, J. (1993) Serum markers of bone type I collagen formation and degradation in metabolic bone disease: correlation with bone histomorphometry. *J. Bone. Miner. Res.* **8**: 127–132.

Eyre, D. R., Koob, T. J., and Van Ness, K. (1984) Quantitation of hydroxypyridinium cross-links in collagen by high-performance liquid chromatography. *Anal. Biochem.* **137**: 380–388.

Faulkner, K. G. (2000) Bone matters: are density increases necessary to reduce fracture risk? *J. Bone Miner. Res.* **15**: 183–187.

Finkelstein, J. S., Mitlak, B. H., and Slovick, D. M. (1997) Osteoporosis. In *Cecils Essentials in Medicine*, Chap. 76, edited by T. E. Andreoli, J. C. Bennett, C. C. J. Carpenter, and F. Plum, Saunders: Philadelphia, PA.

Fiore, C. E., Pennisi, P., Ciffo, F., Scebba, C., Amico, A., and Di Fazzio, S. (1998) Immobilization-dependent bone collagen breakdown appears to increase with time: evidence for a lack of a new bone equilibrium in response to reduced load during prolonged bed rest. *Horm. Metab. Res.* **31**: 31–36.

Fortney, S. M., Schneider, V. S., and Greenleaf, J. E. (1996) The physiology of bed rest. In *Handbook of Physiology,* Section 4: *Environmental Physiology*, edited by M. J. Fregly and C. M. Blatteis, Oxford University Press, New York, Vol. **2**, Chap. 39, pp. 889–939.

Frost, H. M. (1995) An overview: spinal tissue vital biomechanics for clinicians. In *Spinal Disorders in Growth and Aging*, edited by H. E. Takahashi, Springer Verlag: Tokyo, pp. 95–126.

Frost, H. M. (1997) Why do marathon runners have less bone than weight lifters? A vital-biomechanical view and explanation. *Bone* **20**: 183–189.

Fukuoka, H., Kiriyama, M., Nishimura, Y., Higurashi, M., Suzuki, Y., and Gunji, A. (1994) Metabolic turnover of bone and peripheral monocyte release of cytokines during short-term bed rest. *Acta Physiol. Scand.* **150**: (Suppl 616): 37–41.

Garnero, P., and Delmas, P. D. (1998) Biochemical markers of bone turnover: applications for osteoporosis. *Endocrinol. Metab. Clin. North Am.* **27**: 303–323.

Gordon, J. E. (1991) *Structures—or Why Things Don't Fall Down*. Penguin Books: London.

Greenleaf, J. E., and Kozlowski, S. (1982) Physiological consequences of reduced physical activity during bed rest. *Exerc. Sports Sci. Rev.* **20**: 83–119.

Grigoriev, A. I., Bugrov, S. A., Bogomolov, V. V., Egorov, A. D., Kozlovskaya, I. B., Pestov, I. D., Polyakov, V. V., and Tarasov, I. K. (1991) Medical results of the Mir year-long mission. *Physiologist* **34**: S44–S48.

Grigoriev, A. I., Morukov, B. V., Oganov, V. S., Rakhmanov, A. S., and Buravkova, L. B. (1992) Effect of exercise and bisphosphonate on mineral balance and bone density during 360 day antiorthostatic hypokinesia. *J. Bone Miner. Res.* **7**: 449–455.

Grigoryeva, L. S., and Kozlovskaya, I. B. (1987) Effects of weightlessness and hypokinesia on velocity and strength properties of human muscles. *Kosm. Biol. Aviakosm. Med.* **21**: 27–30.

Groenveld, E. H. J., and Burger, E. H. (2000) Bone morphogenetic protein in human bone regeneration. *Eur. J. Endocrinol.* **142**: 9–21.

Hansson, T. H., Roos, B. O., Nachemson, A. (1975) Development of osteopenia in the fourth lumbar vertebra during prolonged bed rest after operation for scoliosis. *Acta Orthoped. Scand.* **46**: 621–636.

Heany, R. P. (1989) Osteoporotic space: an hypothesis. *J. Bone Miner. Res.* **6**: 1–13.

Hofbauer, L. C., and Khosla, S. (1999) Androgen effects on bone metabolism: recent progress and controversies. *Eur. J. Endocrinol.* **140**: 271–286.

Howard, A. D., Berger, J., Familletti, P., and Udenfriend, S. (1987) Characterization of the phosphatidylinositol-glycan membrane anchor of human placental alkaline phosphatase. *Proc. Natl. Acad. Sci. USA* **84**: 6055–6059.

Ingram, R. T., Clarke, B. L., Fisher, L. W., and Fitzpatrick, L. A. (1993) Distribution of noncollagenous proteins in the matrix of adult human bone: evidence of anatomic and functional heterogeneity. *J. Bone Min. Res.* **8**: 1019–1029.

Johnson, P. C., Leach, C. S., and Rambaut, P. C. (1973) Estimates of fluid and energy balances of Apollo 17. *Aerospace Med.* **44**: 1227–1230.

Jones, D. B., Leivseth, G., and Tenbosch, J. (1995) Mechano-reception in osteoblast-like cells. *Biochem. Cell. Biol.* **73**: 525–534.

Kabel, J., van Rietbergen, B., Dalstra, M., Odgaard, A., and Huiskes, R. (1999) The role of an effective isotropic tissue modulus in the elastic properties of cancellous bone. *J. Biomech.* **32**: 673–680.

Kamel, S., Brazier, M., Neri, V., Picard, C., Samson, L., Desmet, G., and Sebert, J. L. (1995) Multiple molecular forms of pyridinoline cross-links excreted in human urine evaluated by chromatographic and immunoassay methods. *J. Bone Miner. Res.* **9**: 1385–1392.

Kaufman, J. J., and Einhorn, T. A. (1993) Ultrasound assessment of bone. *J. Bone Miner. Res.* **8**: 517–525.

Kleerekoper, M., Villanueva, A. R., Stanciu, J., Rao, D. S., and Parfitt, A. M. (1985) The role of three-dimensional trabecular microstructure in the pathogenesis of vertebral compression fractures. *Calcif. Tissue Int.* **37**: 594–597.

Krall, E. A., and Dawson-Hughes, B. (1993) Heritable and life-style determinants of bone mineral density. *J. Bone Miner. Res.* **8**: 1–9.

Krane, S. M., Kantrowitz, F. G., Byrne, M., Pinnell, S. R., and Singer, F. R. (1977) Urinary excretion of hydroxylysine and its glycosides as an index of collagen degradation. *J. Clin. Invest.* **59**: 819–827.

Krasnoff, J., and Painter, P. (1999) The physiological consequences of bed rest and inactivity. *Adv. Ren. Replace. Ther.* **6**: 124–132.

Krølner, B., and Toft, B. (1983) Vertebral bone loss: an unheeded side effect of therapeutic bed rest. *Clin. Sci.* **4**: 537–540.

Krupina, T. N., Tizul, A. Y., Kuzman, M. P., and Tsyganova, N. I. (1982) Clinico-physiological changes in man during long-term antiorthostatic hypokinesia. *Aviat. Space Environ. Med.* **16**: 40–45.

LeBlanc, A. D., Schneider, V. S., Evans, H. J., Engelbretson, D. A., and Krebs, J. M. (1990) Bone mineral loss and recovery after 17 weeks of bed rest. *J. Bone Miner. Res.* **5**: 843–850.

LeBlanc, A., Schneider, V., Spector, E., Evans, H., Rowe, R., Lane, H., Demers, L., and Lipton, A. (1995) Calcium absorption, endogenous secretion and endocrine changes during and after long-term bed rest. *Bone* **16**: 301S–304S.

LeBlanc, A., Shackelford, L., and Schneider, V. (1998) Future human bone research in space. *Bone* **22**: 113S–116S.

Lockwood, D. R., Vogel, J. M., Schneider, V. S., and Hulley, S. B. (1975) Effect of diphosphate EHDP on bone mineral metabolism during prolonged bed rest. *J. Clin. Endocrinol. Metab.* **41**: 533–541.

Lutwak, L., Whedon, G. D., Lachance, P. A., Reid, J. M., and Lipscomb, H. S. (1969) *J. Clin. Endocrinol.* **29**: 1140–1156.

Mack, P. B., LaChance, P. A., Vose, G. P., and Vogt, F. B. (1967) Bone demineralization of foot and hand of Gemini-Titan IV, V and VII astronauts during orbital flight. *Am. J. Roentgenol. Rad. Ther. Nucl. Med.* **100**: 503–511.

Mazess, R. B., and Whedon, G. D. (1983) Immobilization and bone. *Calcif. Tissue Int.* **35**: 265–267.

Miyamoto, A., Shigematsu, T., Fukunaga, T., Kawakami, K., Mukai, C., and Sekiguchi, C. (1998) Medical baseline data collection on bone and muscle change with space flight. *Bone* **22**: 79S–82S.

Morey-Holton, E. R., Schnoes, H. K., DeLuca, H. F., Phelps, M. E., Klein, R. F., (1988) Nissenson, R. H., and Arnaud, C. D. Vitamin D metabolites and bioactive parathyroid hormone levels during Spacelab 2. *Aviat. Space Environ. Med.* **59**: 1038–1041.

Moris, M., Peretz, A., Tjeka, R., Negaban, N., Wouters, M., and Bergmann, P. (1995) Quantitative ultrasound bone measurements: normal values and comparison with bone mineral density by dual x-ray absorptiometry. *Calcif. Tissue Int.* **57**: 6–10.

Moss, M. L. (1991) Bone as a connected cellular network: modeling and testing. In *Topics in Biomechanical Engineering*, edited by G. Ross, Pergamon: New York, pp. 117–119.

Mundy, G., Garrett, R., Harris, S., Chan, J., Chen, D., Rossini, G., Boyce, B., Zhao, M., and Gutierrez, G. (1999) Stimulation of bone formation in vitro and in rodents by statins. *Science* **286**: 1946–1949.

Nishimura, Y., Fukuoka, H., Kiriyama, M., Suzuki, Y., Oyama, K., Ikawa, S., Higurashi, M., and Gunji, A. (1994) Bone turnover and calcium metabolism during 20 days bed rest in young healthy males and females. *Acta Physiol. Scand.* **150**(Suppl 616): 27–35.

Nordin, B. E. C. (1997) Calcium and osteoporosis. *Nutrition* **13**: 664–686.

Oganov, V. S., Cann, C. E., Rakhmanov, A. S. and Ternovoy, S. K. (1990) A computer tomographic investigation of the musculoskeletal system of the spine in humans after long-term space flight. *Kosm. Biol. Aviakosmich. Med.* **24**: 20–21.

Oganov, V. S., Rakhmanov, A. S., Novikov, V. E., Zatsepin, S. T., Rodionova, S. S., Cann, C. (1991) The state of human bone tissue during space flight. *Acta Astronautica* **23**: 129–133.

Ott, S. M. (1993) When bone mass fails to predict bone failure. *Calcif. Tissue Int.* **53**: S7–S13.

Palle, S., Vico, L., Bourrin, S., and Alexandre, C. (1992) Bone tissue response to four-month antiorthostatic bedrest: a bone histomorphometric study. *Calcif. Tissue Int.* **51**: 189–194.

Palumbo, C., Palazzini, S., and Marotti, G. (1990) Morphological study of intercellular functions during osteocyte differentiation. *Bone* **11**: 401–406.

Parfitt, A. M. (1994) Osteonal and hemiosteonal remodeling: the spatial and temporal framework for signal traffic in adult human bone. *J. Cell. Biochem.* **55**: 273–286.

Patel, A. N., Razzak, Z. A., and Dastur, D. K. (1969) Disuse atrophy of human skeletal muscles. *Arch. Neurol.* **20**: 413–421.

Pinnell, S. R., Fox, R., and Krane, S. M. (1971) Human collagens: differences in glycosylated hydroxylysines in skin and bone. *Biochim. Biophys. Acta* **229**: 119–122.

Pruitt, L. S., Jackson, R. D., Bartels, R. L., and Lehnhard, H. J. (1992) Weight-training effects on bone mineral density in early postmenopausal women. *J. Bone Miner. Res.* **7**: 179–185.

Raab, D. M., Crenchaw, T. D., Kimmel, D. B., and Smith, E. L. (1991) A histomorphometric study of the cortical bone activity during increased weight-bearing exercise. *J. Bone Miner. Res.* **6**: 741–749.

Rambaut, P. C., Leach, C. S., and Johnson, P. C. (1975) Calcium and phosphorus change of the Apollo 17 crew members. *Nutr. Metab.* **18**: 62–69.

Reich, K. M., Gay, C. V., and Frangos, J. A.(1990) Fluid shear stress as a mediator of osteoblast cyclic adenosine monophosphate production. *J. Cell. Physiol.* **143**: 100–104.

Risteli, L., and Risteli, J.(1993) Biochemical markers of bone metabolism. *Ann. Med.* **25**: 385–393.

Roux, W. (1895) *Gesammelte Abhandlung über die Entwicklungsmechanik der Organismen*. Vols. I and II, W. Engelmann: Leipzig.

Rubin, C. T., and Lanyon, L. E. (1987) Osteoregulatory nature of mechanical stimuli: function as a determinant for adaptive bone remodeling. *J. Orthop. Res.* **5**: 300–310.

Saltin, B., Blomqvist, G., Mitchell, J. H., Johnson, R. L., Wildenthal, K., and Chapman, C. B. (1968) Response to exercise after bed rest and after training: A longitudinal study of adaptive changes in oxygen transport and body composition. *Circulation* **38**: VII-1-78.

Sargeant, A. J., Davies, C. T. M., Edwards, R. H. T., Maunder, C., and Young, A. (1977) Functional and structural changes after disuse of human muscle. *Clin. Sci. Mol. Med.* **52**: 337–342.

Sauren, Y. M. H. F., Mieremet, R. H. P., Groot, C. G., and Scherft, J. P. (1992) An electron microscopic study on the presence of proteoglycans in the mineralized matrix of rat and human compact lamellar bone. *Anat. Rec.* **232**: 36–44.

Sawin, C. F. (1998) Biomedical investigations conducted in support of the extended duration orbiter medical project. *Texas Med.* **94**: 56–68.

Schneider, V. S. (1991) Attempts to prevent bone mineral loss during prolonged bedrest. Washington, DC: NASA SP-452, 85 pp.

Schneider, V., Oganov, V., LeBlanc, A., Rakhmanov, A., Bakulin, A., Grigoriev, A., and Varonin, L. (1992) Space flight bone loss and change in fat and lean body mass. *J. Bone Miner. Res.* **117**: S122.

Schnitzler, C. M. (1993) Bone quality: a determinant for certain risk factors for bone fragility. *Calcif. Tissue Int.* **53**: S27–S31.

Shackelford, L. C., LeBlanc, A., Feiveson, A., and Oganov, V. (1999) Bone loss in space: Shuttle/MIR experience and bed rest countermeasure program. In *Proceedings of the First Biennial Space Biomedical Investigators' Workshop*, NASA / USRA, p. 235.

Skerry, T. M. (1997) Mechanical loading and bone: what sort of exercise is beneficial to the skeleton? *Bone* **20**: 179–181.

Smith, M. C. Jr., Rambaut, P. C., Vogel, J. M., and Whittle, M. W. (1977) Bone mineral measurement—Experiment M078. In *Biomedical Results from Skylab*, edited by R. S. Johnston and L. F. Dietlein, Washington, DC: NASA SP-377, pp. 183–190.

Smith. S. M., Nillen, J. L., Leblanc, A., Lipton, A., Demers, L. M., Lane, H. W., and Leach, C. S. (1998) Collagen cross-link excretion during space flight and bed rest. *J. Clin. Endocrinol. Metab.* **83**: 3584–3591.

Smith, S. M., Wastney, M. E., Morukov, B.V., Larina, I. M., Nyquist, L. E., Abrams, S. A., Taran, E. N., Shih, C. Y., Nillen, J. L., Davi-Street, J. E., Rice, B. L., Lane, H. W. (1999) Calcium metabolism before, during, and after a 3-mo spaceflight: kinetic and biochemical changes. *Am. J. Physiol. Regulatory Integrative Comp. Physiol.* **277**: R1–R10.

Sone, T., Imai, Y., Tomomitsu, T., and Fukunaga, M. (1998) Calcaneus as a site for the assessment of bone mass. *Bone* **22**: 155S–157S.

Takano, Y., Turner, C. H., Owan, I., Martin, R. B., Lau, S. T., Forwood, M. R., and Burr, D B. (1999) Elastic anisotropy and collagen orientation of osteonal bone are dependent on the mechanical strain distribution. *J. Orthop. Res.* **17**: 59–66.

Tothill, P. (1989) Methods of bone mineral measurement. *Physiol. Med. Biol.* **34**: 543–572.

Triffitt, J. T. (1987) The special proteins of bone tissue. *Clin. Sci.* **72**: 399–408.

Turner, C. H. (1999) Site-specific skeletal effects of exercise: importance of interstitial fluid pressure. *Bone* **24**: 161–162.

Van der Weil, H. E., Lips, P., Nauta, J., Netelenbos, J. C., and Hazenberg, G. J. (1991) Biochemical parameters of bone turnover during ten days of bed rest and subsequent mobilization. *Bone Miner.* **13**: 123–129.

Vico, L., Chappard, D., Alexandre, C., Palle, S., Minaire, P., Riffat, G., Morukov, B., and Rakhmanov, S. (1987) Effects of a 120-day period of bed-rest on bone mass and bone cell activities in man: attempts at countermeasure. *Bone Miner.* **2**: 383–394.

Vogel, G. (1999) Capturing the promise of youth. *Science* **286**: 2238–2239.

Vogel, J. M., Wasnich, R. D., and Ross, P. D. (1988) The clinical relevance of calcaneus bone mineral measurements: a review. *Bone Miner.* **5**: 35–58.

Vogel, J. M., and Whittle, M. W. (1976a) Bone mineral changes: the second manned Skylab mission. *Aviat. Space Environ. Med.* **47**: 396–400.

Vogel, J. M., and Whittle, M. W. (1976b) Bone mineral content changes in the Skylab astronauts. *Am. J. Roentgenol. Rad. Ther. Nucl. Med.* **126**: 1296–1297.

Vose, G. P.(1974) Review of roentgenographic bone demineralization studies of the Gemini space flights. *Am. J. Roentgenol. Rad. Ther. Nucl. Med.* **121**: 1–4.

Wang, N., Butler, J. P., and Ingber, D. E. (1993) Mechanotransduction across the cell surface and through the cytoskeleton. *Science* **260**: 1124–1127.

Weinbaum, S., Cowin, S. C., and Zeng, Y. (1994) A model for the excitation of osteocytes by mechanical loading-induced bone fluid shear stresses. *J. Biomech.* **27**: 339–360.

Whedon, G. D., Lutwak, L., Reid, J., Rambaut, P., Whittle, M., Smith, M., and Leach, C. (1975) Mineral and nitrogen balance study, results of metabolic observations on Skylab II 28-day orbital mission. *Acta Astronautica* **2**: 297–309.

White, R. J. (1998) Weightlessness and the human body. *Sci. Am.* **279**: 39–43.

Wolff, J. D. (1892) *Das Gesetz der Transformation der Knochen.* A. Hirschwald, Berlin.

Zerwekh, J. E., Ruml, L. A., Gottschalk, F., and Pak, C. Y. C. (1998) The effects of twelve weeks of bed rest on bone histology, biochemical markers of bone turnover, and calcium homeostasis in eleven normal subjects. *J. Bone Miner. Res.* **13**: 1594–1601.

CHAPTER 8

Bed Rest Muscular Atrophy

John E. Greenleaf

*Laboratory for Human Environmental Physiology, NASA,
Ames Research Center, Moffett Field, California, USA*

> For if the whole body is rested much
> more than is usual, there is no immediate
> increase in strength. In fact, should a long
> period of inactivity be followed by a
> sudden return to exercise, there will be an
> obvious deterioration….The same is true
> of the teeth and of the eyes, and in fact of
> every part of the body.
>
> *Hippocrates*

INTRODUCTION

A major debilitating response from prolonged bed rest (BR) is muscle atrophy, defined as a "decrease in size of a part of tissue after full development has been attained: a wasting away of tissue as from disuse, old age, injury or disease" (*Webster's New International Dictionary*, 3rd ed., 1986, s.v. "muscle atrophy"). Part of the complicated mechanism for the dizziness, increased body instability, and exaggerated gait in patients who arise immediately after BR may be a result of not only foot pain, but also of muscular atrophy and associated reduction in lower limb strength. Also, there seems to be a close association between muscle atrophy and bone atrophy (Chapter 7; Rodahl et al., 1967). A discussion of many facets of the total BR homeostatic syndrome has been published (Fortney et al., 1996).

The old adage that use determines form which promotes function of bone (Wolff's law) also applies to those people exposed to prolonged BR (without exercise training) in whom muscle atrophy is a consistent finding (Fortney et al., 1996; LeBlanc et al., 1992). An extreme case involved a 16-year-old boy who was ordered

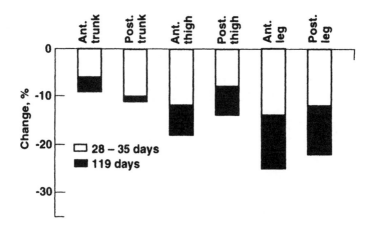

Figure 8.1 Mean percent changes in muscle mass from the trunk, thigh, and leg at 28–35 days and 119 days of BR. (From LeBlanc et al., 1992, 1997 magnetic resonance imaging-pixels; Ellis et al., 1993 ultrasound-cm.)

to bed by his mother in 1932: after 50 years in bed he had "a lily-white frame with limbs as thin as the legs of a ladder-back chair" (Associated Press, 1982). These findings emphasize the close relationship between muscle atrophy and bone atrophy (Fortney et al., 1966; LeBlanc et al., 1997; Treharne, 1981). In addition to loss of muscle mass during deconditioning, there is a significant loss of muscle strength and a decrease in protein synthesis. Because the decreases in force (strength) are proportionately greater than those in fiber size or muscle cross-sectional area (Berg et al., 1991), other contributory factors must be involved; muscle fiber dehydration may be important (Bosco et al., 1968).

MACRO-ATROPHY

The extensor muscles that extend a joint in ambulatory people are used to maintain the upright (sitting or standing) posture to counteract the force of gravity. Some such back muscles are located in the posterior trunk (semispinalis, longissimus, iliocostalis), anterior thigh (knee extensors—quadriceps femoris), and posterior leg (ankle extensors—soleus, gastrocnemius). A decrease in muscle mass in those groups during deconditioning, as measured from magnetic resonance imaging (MRI) sections, occurs in both flexor and extensor muscles: by 8% in the calf after 24 hr of BR (Conley et al., 1996), by 3% within the first 7 days of BR (Ferrando et al., 1995), by 5% within 14 days of BR (LeBlanc et al., 1992), by 5% to 10% by 20–28 days of BR (Akima et al., 1997; Greenleaf et al., 1994b); muscle mass continues to decline thereafter to 112 days of BR (Figure 8.1). In general, the rate of decrease in muscle mass by 35 days of BR is greater than that to 112 days of BR in the trunk, thigh, and leg. Also, circumferences of the arm, chest, waist, thigh, and calf decrease by 0.1% to 3.4% during BR from 9 to 252 days (Greenleaf and Kozlowski, 1982); loss of fat and water from muscle likely contribute to this volume contraction (LeBlanc et al., 1987).

Magnetic resonance imaging is useful for measuring the changes in muscle size and composition that accompany BR-deconditioning. In addition to loss of fat and water, the contrast in MR images arises from many other factors such as concentration and conformation of macromolecules. Typical MR images used to estimate changes in muscle volume are designated T1—weighted as brightness of the image intensity—which is inversely related to the T1 relaxation time of the signal and characterizes the exponential rate of recovery of the magnetization induced by placing tissue in a magnetic field. A second MRI parameter (T2) characterizes the rate of decay of the MR signal; it is particularly sensitive to and generally increases in proportion to tissue water content. T1 relaxation is transfer of energy to adjacent nuclei and similar resonant frequencies; whereas T2 relaxation involves interaction between excited nuclei and magnetic fields with no energy loss, thereby increasing the probability of such interactions and shorter relaxation times (Adams et al., 1992). To the extent that response of proton $[H^+]$ T2 relaxation times reflect fluid shifts from water bound to the shell of macromolecules and those of free unbound water (Fullerton et al., 1982), it is surprising that MRI scans indicate that the decrease in limb muscle cross-sectional areas (thus their volume) is not caused at least in part by fluid loss. Both LeBlanc et al. (1986) and Conley et al. (1996) reported no significant change in T2 values from resting leg muscle MRI scans during deconditioning in rats and humans. These findings are difficult to reconcile with the well-established decreases in total body water, plasma volume, and limb size and muscle volume that occur with prolonged BR (Fortney et al., 1996) (since striated muscle is about 80% water). Adams et al. (1992) have reported that T2 is increased as a function of exercise load, and that the increase in muscle volume during exercise is mainly a result of influx and binding of water. If this is so, why is there not efflux of water from muscle during deconditioning?

Thus, this macro-muscle atrophy begins within the first few days of BR in the absence of exercise training and reaches 20% to 30% by 17 weeks in both flexor and especially extensor leg muscles.

MUSCULAR STRENGTH

Maximal static and isokinetic muscular strengths decrease in virtually every major muscle group from the first week of BR without remedial exercise training (Bloomfield, 1997; Greenleaf et al., 1983; Krasnoff and Painter, 1999). Static maximal strength losses can be 5% to 9% (upper extremities) and 1% to 14% (lower extremities) during 44 days of BR, but they continue decreasing to 26% to 48% (upper) and 36% to 58% (lower) from 63 days to 95 days of BR (Figure 8.2). In addition to significant loss of contractile function because of muscle atrophy, it may be more difficult "psychologically" to increase the tension to perform a maximal strength test after

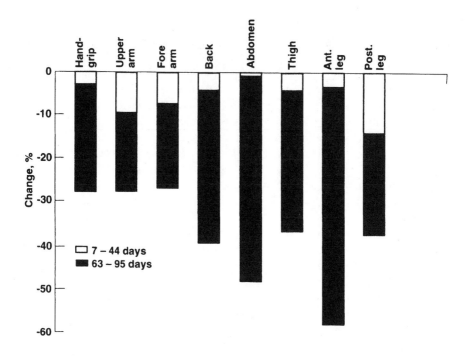

Figure 8.2 Mean percent changes in maximal (static) muscular strength during 7 to 44 days and 63 to 95 days of BR. (From Greenleaf et al., 1983; 63–95 day data from Yeremin et al., 1969.)

extended BR-deconditioning, so the actual losses with prolonged BR could even be greater.

Maximal isokinetic muscular strength does not decrease in all major muscle groups during BR without remedial exercise; the decrements seem to be localized in the lower extremities (Greenleaf et al., 1994a; LeBlanc et al., 1992). LeBlanc et al. (1992) found that isokinetic strength (performed at a velocity of $60°·sec^{-1}$) decreased progressively over 112 days of BR (Figure 8.3): more so in the thighs and legs (from 11 to 31%) than in the arms (from +4 to −6%), and more so during the first 35 days (from 10 to 25%) than at 112 days where the additional lower extremity losses increased by only 1 to 8%. Greenleaf et al. (1994a) partially confirmed these findings in five men over 26 days of BR where there was no significant change in peak torque ($100°·sec^{-1}$) for shoulder abduction and adduction, but significant decrease in knee flexion strength. Isotonic aerobic exercise training and isokinetic strength training daily during 28 days of BR (Figure 8.4) resulted in no change or increases, respectively, in peak torque for right knee extension when compared with the progressively decreasing torque with no exercise training (Greenleaf et al., 1989). Bamman et al. (1997) also reported complete restoration of plantar flexor angle-specific torque and average power at all velocities after 14 days of 6° head-down BR with multi-set, constant resistance, concentric/eccentric plantar

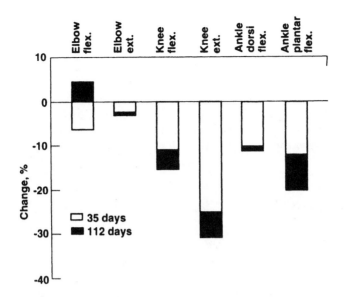

Figure 8.3 Mean percent changes in isokinetic (dynamic) muscular strength at $60° \cdot \sec^{-1}$ after 35 days and 112 days of BR (* $p < 0.05$ from zero). (From LeBlanc et al., 1992.)

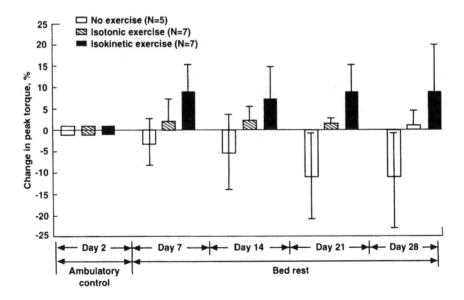

Figure 8.4 Mean ($\pm$SE) percent changes in peak torque for right knee extension during 29 days of $-6°$.

flexion–extension work to fatigue. Also, strength losses were similar for eccentric (lengthening) and concentric (shortening) muscle actions that were independent of contraction velocity, suggesting that selective atrophy of specific fiber types did not occur (Dudley et al., 1989).

Thus, in contrast to the general decrease in static strength in both upper and lower extremity muscle groups, these isokinetic strength responses were of lesser magnitude and the decrements were located mainly in muscles of the lower extremities. Compared with ambulatory muscular deconditioning, there is a greater loss in both static and dynamic strength in relation to muscle cross-sectional area or volume during BR. Perhaps this discrepancy results in part from the preferential loss of water from deconditioned muscles.

MICRO-ATROPHY

The decrease in gross muscle size during prolonged BR is a reflection of muscle water content, as well as other cellular events in its fat, connective tissue, and fiber content, the latter being the more pliable. The more frequently studied muscles are the soleus (an ankle plantar flexor) and the vastus lateralis (a knee extensor)—those that help maintain the erect posture and also respond more readily to deconditioning.

After 17 days of 6° head-down BR the soleus muscle fibers (slow Type I myosin heavy chain, MHC) in men exhibited a significant decrease in peak isometric force (P_0) of 11% to 13% (Widrick et al., 1997, 1998); also, Type I fiber unloaded shortening velocity (V_0) at peak power output was increased by 13% to 34%. Thus, the increased velocity facilitates maintenance of power (force × velocity) as atrophy reduces force (Riley et al., 1998). Fiber-packing density of the thick myofilaments was unchanged with BR, but thin-filament (actin) density was decreased by 16% to 24% (Riley et al., 1998; Widrick et al., 1997). The correlation (r^2) between increased V_0 and decreased thin-filament density was 0.62; a 1% decrease in filament density increased V_0 by about 10% (Riley et al., 1998). These findings lead to the hypothesis that changes in the geometry between thick and thin filaments may be associated with the elevated V_0, because fewer filaments would increase interfilament spacing resulting in earlier cross-bridge detachment, thereby increasing velocity.

In general, the vastus lateralis muscle responds similarly to the soleus even after somewhat longer periods (37 days to 42 days) of BR deconditioning. The specific tension ratio (P_0/cross-sectional area, CSA) decreased by 32% to 48%, and was associated with decreased myofibrillar protein content which is primarily related to a decreased number of force-generating cross-bridges (Larsson et al., 1996). The 13% decrease in CSA increased the P_0/CSA ratio which should be considered when compared with only the P_0 values cited previously for the soleus muscle. The V_0 in Type I MHC isoforms decreased by 49% in two of three subjects and was associated with changes in myosin light chain isoform composition. Andersen et al. (1999) have reported altered MHC gene expression leading to unusual combinations of mRNA and MHC isoforms, but there were no commensurate changes to the protein level alone suggesting an increased number of muscle fibers in a transitional state. Observation of gross structural anatomy of muscle after 30 days of BR in men (Hikida et al.,

1989) and 5 months of close confinement in male mongrel dogs (Nazar et al., 1993) reveals similar fiber disorganization, degeneration, and decreased mitochondrial density, which must contribute to decreased muscular function. Essentially all of the latter anatomical aberrations were restored to normal after the dogs were released from confinement.

PROPRIOCEPTIVE REFLEXES AND LIMB TRACKING

Proprioceptive reflexes (from recorded bioelectric activity of latent periods) and muscle tone were measured in six young men after 62 days of horizontal BR without and with 1,100 kcal·day^{-1} of physical exercise (Cherepakhin, 1968). Although muscle tone decreased during the no-exercise phase, there were no significant changes in the mandibular, biceps, triceps, shoulder, knee, or Achilles reflexes in either the exercise or nonexercise phases: duration of the reflex latent periods was proportional to path length; for example, mandibular was 5 msec and Achilles was 34 msec.

Another facet of proprioception was measured in 19 men—36±4 yr, with no exercise (NOE) and isotonic (ITE) and isokinetic (IKE) leg exercise training during BR—after 30 days of −6° head-down BR (Bernauer et al., 1994). Only the IKE group performed proprioceptive training (1 min of leg tracking while viewing a vertically oscillating bar on a biofeedback computer screen) daily during BR; the NOE and ITE groups performed the tracking test only weekly. After BR, there were no significant changes in tracking with NOE, but there were significant increases in the two exercise groups (ITE and IKE). Thus, 30 days of BR deconditioning does not appear to compromise these proprioceptive reflexes or leg tracking.

POSTURAL CONTROL AFTER BED REST

Ambulation and maintenance of body balance are usually impaired after prolonged BR (Davis, Horwood, and De Jong, 1997; Gretebeck and Greenleaf, 1999; Haines, 1974). Upon standing after BR there is usually pain from the plantar foot, in the lower limb joints, and in muscles, especially those in the upper back and neck (Haines, 1974); enhanced postural instability measured by increased electromyographic activity (Davis et al., 1997); and impaired rail walking and balance (especially with eyes open) compounded by increased pre-syncopal episodes (Gretebeck and Greenleaf, 1999; Haines, 1974). Daily isotonic or isometric exercise training during BR, with increased leg extension strength (Greenleaf et al., 1989) and unchanged or increased proprioception tracking (Bernauer et al., 1994) did not influence or ameliorate this impaired postural ambulation or control after BR.

Recovery of postural control after BR occurs after 3–4 days of ambulation, and balance test results return to normal faster with eyes open (Haines, 1974).

Presyncopal signs and symptoms (tendency to faint with decreased cerebral blood flow) may be involved (Drozdova and Nesterenko, 1969).

REFERENCES

Adams, G. R., Duvoisin, M. R., and Dudley, G. A. (1992) Magnetic resonance imaging and electromyography as indexes of muscle function. *J. Appl. Physiol.* **73**: 1578–1583.

Akima, H., Kuno, S., Suzuki, Y., Gunji, A., and Fukunaga, T. (1997) Effects of 20 days of bed rest on physiological cross-sectional area of human thigh and leg muscles evaluated by magnetic resonance imaging. *J. Gravit. Physiol.* **4**: S15–S21.

Andersen, J. L., Gruschy-Knudsen, T., Sandri, C., Larsson, L., and Schiaffino, S. (1999) Bed rest increases the amount of mismatched fibers in human skeletal muscle. *J. Appl. Physiol.* **86**: 455–460.

Associated Press. (1982) Puzzling illness keeps man in bed 50 years. *San Jose Mercury News*, May 26, p. 12A.

Bamman, M. M., Hunter, G. R., Stevens, B. R., Guilliams, M. E., and Greenisen, M. C. (1997) Resistance exercise prevents plantar flexor deconditioning during bed rest. *Med. Sci. Sports Exerc.* **29**: 1462–1468.

Berg, H. E., Dudley, G. A., Häggmark, T., Ohlsen, H., and Tesch, P. A. (1991) Effects of lower limb unloading on skeletal muscle mass and function in humans. *J. Appl. Physiol.* **70**: 1882–1885.

Bernauer, E. M., Walby, W. F., Ertl, A. C., Dempster, P. T., Bond, M., and Greenleaf, J. E. (1994) Knee-joint proprioception during 30-day 6° head-down bed rest with isotonic and isokinetic exercise training. *Aviat. Space Environ. Med.* **65**: 1110–1115.

Bloomfield, S. A. (1997) Changes in musculoskeletal structure and function with prolonged bed rest. *Med. Sci. Sports Exerc.* **29**: 197–206.

Bosco, J. S., Terjung, R. L., and Greenleaf, J. E. (1968) Effects of progressive hypohydration on maximal isometric muscular strength. *J. Sports Med. Phys. Fitness* **8**: 81–86.

Cherepakin, M. A. (1968) Effect of prolonged bedrest on muscle tone and proprioceptive reflexes in man. *Kosm. Biol. Med.* **2**: 43–47.

Conley, M. S., Foley, J. M., Ploutz-Snyder, L. L., Meyer, R. A., and Dudley, G.A. (1996) Effect of acute head-down tilt on skeletal muscle cross-sectional area and proton transverse relaxation time. *J. Appl. Physiol.* **81**: 1572–1577.

Davis, J. E., Horwood, K. E., and DeJong, G. K. (1997) Effects of exercise during head-down bed rest on postural control. *Aviat. Space Environ. Med.* **68**: 392–395.

Drozdova, N. T., and Nesterenko, O. N. (1969) State of the visual analyzer during hypodynamia. In *Problemy Kosmicheskoy Biologii*, edited by A. M. Genin and P. A. Sorokin, Nauka Press: Moscow, **13**: 189–191.

Dudley, G. A., Duvoisin, M. R., Convertino, V. A., and Buchanan, P. (1989) Alterations of the in vivo torque-velocity relationship of human skeletal muscle following 30 days exposure to simulated microgravity. *Aviat. Space Environ. Med.* **60**: 659–663.

Ellis S., Kirby, L. C., and Greenleaf, J. E. (1993) Lower extremity muscle thickness during 30-day 6° head-down bed rest with isotonic and isokinetic exercise training. *Aviat. Space Environ. Med.* **64**: 1011–1015.

Ferrando, A. A., Stuart, C. A., Brunder, D. G., and Hillman, G. R. (1995) Magnetic resonance imaging quantitation of changes in muscle volume during 7 days of strict bed rest. *Aviat. Space. Environ. Med.* **66**: 976–981.

Fortney, S. M., Schneider, V. S., and Greenleaf, J. E. (1996) The physiology of bed rest. In *Handbook of Physiology*: Section 4: *Environmental Physiology*, edited by M. J. Fregly and C. M. Blatteis, Oxford University Press: New York, Vol. 2, Chap. 39, pp. 889–939.

Fullerton, G. D., Potter, J. L., and Dornbluth, N. C. (1982) NMR relaxation of protons in tissues and other macromolecular water solutions. *Magn. Reson. Imaging* **1**: 209–228.

Greenleaf, J. E., Bernauer, E. M., Ertl, A. C., Bulbulian, R., and Bond, M. (1994a) Isokinetic strength and endurance during 30-day 6° head-down bed rest with isotonic and isokinetic exercise training. *Aviat. Space Environ. Med.* **65**: 45–50.

Greenleaf, J. E., Bernauer, E. M., Ertl, A. C., Trowbridge, T. S., and Wade, C. E. (1989) Work capacity during 30 days of bed rest with isotonic and isokinetic exercise training. *J. Appl. Physiol.* **67**: 1820–1826.

Greenleaf, J. E., and Kozlowski, S. (1982) Physiological consequences of reduced physical activity during bed rest. In *Exerc. Sport. Sci. Rev.* **10**, edited by R. L. Terjung, Franklin Institute Press: Philadelphia, PA, pp. 84–119.

Greenleaf, J. E., Lee, P. L., Ellis, S., Selzer, R. H., and Ortendahl, D. A. (1994b) Leg muscle volume during 30-day 6-degree head-down bed rest with isotonic and isokinetic exercise training. Moffett Field, CA, NASA TM-4580, 8 pp.

Greenleaf, J. E, Van Beaumont, W., Convertino, V. A., and Starr, J. C. (1983) Handgrip and general muscular strength and endurance during prolonged bed rest with isometric and isotonic leg exercise training. *Aviat. Space Environ. Med.* **54**: 696–700.

Gretebeck, R. J., and Greenleaf, J. E. (2000) Utility of ground-based simulations of weightlessness. In *Nutrition in Space Flight and Weightlessness Models*, edited by H. W. Lane and D. A. Schoeller, CRC Press: Boca Raton, FL, pp. 69–96.

Haines, R. F. (1974) Effect of bed rest and exercise on body balance. *J. Appl. Physiol.* **36**: 323–327.

Hikida, R. S., Gollnick, P. D., Dudley, G. A., Convertino, V. A., and Buchanan, P. (1989) Structural and metabolic characteristics of human skeletal muscle following 30 days of simulated microgravity. *Aviat. Space Environ. Med.* **60**: 664–670.

Krasnoff, J., and Painter, P. (1999) The physiological consequences of bed rest and inactivity. *Adv. Ren. Replace. Ther.* **6**: 124–132.

Larsson, L., Li, X., Berg, H. E., and Frontera, W. R. (1996) Effects of removal of weight-bearing function on contractility and myosin isoform composition in single human skeletal muscle cells. *Pflügers Arch.* **432**: 320–328.

LeBlanc, A., Evans, H., Schonfeld, E., Ford, J., Marsh, C., Schneider, V., and Johnson, P. (1986) Relaxation times of normal and atrophied muscle. *Med. Phys.* **13**: 514–517.

LeBlanc, A., Evans, H., Schonfeld, E., Ford, J., Schneider, V., Jhingran, S., and Johnson, P. (1987) Changes in nuclear magnetic resonance (T2) relaxation of limb tissue with bed rest. *Magn. Reson. Med.* **4**: 487–492.

LeBlanc, A., Rowe, R., Evans, H., West, S., Shackelford, L., and Schneider, V. (1997) Muscle atrophy during long duration bed rest. *Int. J. Sports Med.* **18**: S283–S334.

LeBlanc, A. D., Schneider, V. S., Evans, H. J., Pientok, C., Rowe, R., and Spector, E. (1992) Regional changes in muscle mass following 17 weeks of bed rest. *J. Appl. Physiol.* **73**: 2172–2178.

Nazar, K., Greenleaf, J. E., Philpott, D., Pohoska, E., Olszewska, K., and Kaciuba-Uscilko, H. (1993) Muscle mitochondrial density after exhaustive exercise in dogs: prolonged restricted activity and retraining. *Aviat. Space Environ. Med.* **64**: 306–313.

Riley, D. A., Bain, J. L. W., Thompson, J. L., Fitts, R. H., Widrick, J. J., Trappe, S. W., Trappe, T. A., and Costill, D. L. (1998) Disproportionate loss of thin filaments in human soleus muscle after 17-day bed rest. *Muscle Nerve* **21**: 1280–1289.

Rodahl, K., Birkhead, N. C., Blizzard, J. J., Issekutz, B. Jr, and Pruett, E. D. R. (1967) Physiological changes during prolonged bed rest. In *Nutrition and Physical Activity*, edited by G. Blix, Almqvist & Wiksells: Uppsala, Sweden, pp. 107–113.

Treharne, R. W. (1981) Review of Wolff's law and its proposed means of operation. *Orthop. Rev.* **10**: 35–47.

Widrick, J. J., Norenberg, K. M., Romatowski, J. G., Blaser, C. A., Karhanek, M., Sherwood, J., Trappe, S.W., Trappe, T. A., Costill, D. L., and Fitts, R. H. (1998) Force-velocity-power and force-pCa relationships of human soleus fibers after 17 days of bed rest. *J. Appl. Physiol.* **85**: 1949–1956.

Widrick, J. J., Romatowski, J. G., Bain, J. L. W., Trappe, S. W., Trappe, T. A., Thompson, J. L., Costill, D. L., Riley, D. A., and Fitts, R. H.(1997) Effect of 17 days of bed rest on peak isometric force and unloaded shortening velocity of human soleus fibers. *Am. J. Physiol. Cell Physiol.* **273**: C1690–C1699.

Yeremin, A. V., Bazhanov, V. V., Marishchuk, V. L., Stepantsov, V. I., and Dzhamgarov, T. T. (1969) Physical conditioning for man under conditions of prolonged hypodynamia. In *Problemy Kosmicheskoy Biologii*, edited by A. M. Genin and P. A. Sorokin, Nauka Press: Moscow **13**: 192–199.

CHAPTER 9

Bed Rest and Orthostatic-Hypotensive Intolerance

Suzanne M. Schneider

Department of Physical Performance and Development,
University of New Mexico, Albuquerque, New Mexico, USA

Teach us to live that we may dread
unnecessary time in bed,
Get people up and we may save
our patients from an early grave.

R. A. J. Asher

RESPONSE VERSUS TOLERANCE

Orthostatic tolerance may be defined as the ability of humans to maintain cerebral perfusion and consciousness upon movement from a supine or sitting position to the upright posture; for example, subjects can stand suddenly or be tilted to the head-up body position. Similar but not identical physiological responses can be induced by positive G_z (head to foot) acceleration or exposure to lower body negative pressure (LBNP). The objective is to suddenly shift blood to the lower body to determine how effectively cardiovascular and neural-hormonal compensatory responses react to maintain blood pressure. In the most precise method for measuring tolerance, individuals would be stressed until they faint (syncope). However, the potential consequences and discomforts of such a test usually prohibit such a procedure so that few investigators actually induce syncope. In a more common approach the subjects are exposed to a given level of stress; for example, head-up tilt for 15 min, and any increases in heart rate or decreases in blood pressure are interpreted as indicators of progress toward syncope. Presumably, the greater the perturbation of heart rate and blood pressure, the closer to "tolerance," i.e., point of unconsciousness.

Another more appropriate approach is to induce a progressively increasing hypotensive stress until pre-determined physiological responses or pre-syncopal symptoms appear. The physiological criteria may include a sudden drop in systolic blood pressure (>25 mmHg·min^{-1}), a sudden drop in heart rate (>15 beats·min^{-1}), or a systolic blood pressure <70 mmHg. The most common pre-syncopal symptoms include light-headedness, stomach awareness or distress, feelings of warmth, tingly skin, and light to profuse sweating. Usually a combination of physiological responses and symptoms occur such that, on different days, the tolerance time to the same orthostatic protocol is reproducible for a given individual. The assumption is that by taking subjects to near fainting, one can determine their tolerance.

This latter pre-syncopal approach is better for estimating orthostatic or hypotensive tolerance than the former measurement of heart rate and blood pressure responses to a given stress. There is considerable variability in individual responses to orthostasis. For example, some subjects are "heart-rate responders" and have a pronounced cardiovascular response similar to that when performing moderately hard aerobic exercise, whereas others may experience pre-syncopal symptoms with very little increase in heart rate. Some individuals have a slow, gradual fall in blood pressure to orthostasis, and others have little change in blood pressure until a sudden precipitous fall in pressure occurs just prior to fainting. With both tilt and LBNP tests there is a low correlation between heart-rate or blood-pressure responses to a sub-tolerance stress as a measure of pre-syncopal limited orthostatic-hypotensive tolerance (Fortney et al., 1996).

ORTHOSTATIC AND HYPOTENSIVE TOLERANCE AFTER BED REST

Duration of Bed Rest

Orthostatic tolerance decreases following even brief exposure (1–4 hr) to horizontal or head-down bed rest (BR) (Butler et al., 1991; Shi et al., 1992; Vogt, 1967; Pannier et al., 1991). Vogt (1967) found reduced head-up tilt (HUT) tolerance (time to pre-syncope), greater increases in heart rate, and a faster decline in blood pressure after only 12 hr of recumbency. After 2 weeks of BR the increase in heart rate upon standing was almost double that seen before BR, and the fall in stroke volume and cardiac output was twice as great (Harper and Lyles, 1988). The degree of intolerance with BR, however, does not appear to be a function of the length of the recumbency. In a 17-week horizontal BR study in which weekly graded LBNP tests were used, marked changes in the hypotensive response occurred after the first week, with no further significant change during the remaining 16 weeks (Lathers and Charles, 1993).

Although deterioration in orthostatic tolerance may occur rapidly, the mechanisms responsible may not remain the same throughout prolonged BR. For example, simply replacing body fluids during the first week may be an effective treatment (Hyatt and West, 1977). However, as BR continues, additional mechanisms such as loss of ability to vasoconstrict or increased heart rate may become significant factors compromising tolerance.

Chair Rest, Hypodynamia, Confined Environments

Orthostatic tolerance is impaired during decreasing levels of physical activity, even without reduction in the hydrostatic gradient in the body. Prolonged sitting or other reduction in activity may result in increased blood pooling in the lower body or delay in the onset of vasoactive reflexes. Increased orthostatic intolerance occurred in subjects who were exposed to prolonged sitting (Convertino, 1991; Sullivan et al., 1985), in subjects who reduced their daily activities sufficiently to reduce their aerobic capacity (Raven et al., 1998), and in ambulatory subjects living in a confined environment (Lamb et al., 1964). Conversely, brief periods of upright sitting exercise during an extended BR-deconditioning period may improve orthostatic-hypotensive responses, but usually did not completely restore tolerance to pre-BR levels (Birkhead et al., 1964; Watenpaugh et al., 1994). However, supine exercise training without simultaneous orthostatic stress was not effective in maintaining orthostatic tolerance (Birkhead et al., 1966; Greenleaf et al., 1989).

Men versus Women

It has been reported that women have a lower orthostatic tolerance than men (Hordinsky et al., 1981; Montgomery et al., 1977; Gottshall, 2000; White et al., 1996; Convertino, 1998) although others have reported that there are no sex diffe-rences (Frey and Hoffler, 1988; Frey et al., 1986; Rhaman et al., 1991; Lightfoot and Tsintgiras, 1995). Part of the discrepancy may derive from the great individual variation in tolerance that exists among men and women, thus making it necessary to evaluate large samples of each population to derive an appropriate conclusion. Potential mechanisms for a lower orthostatic tolerance in women compared to men may be related to their smaller blood volume, a reduced ability to increase heart rate in response to falling arterial pressure (reduced sensitivity of their carotid-cardiac baroreflex), a higher baseline heart rate and thus less cardiac reserve due to a lower vagal activity and/or an enhanced cardiac beta-adrenergic sensitivity), a greater decline in cardiac output during orthostasis due to enhanced blood pooling in splan-chnic regions (Montgomery, 1977), and/or to a blunted release of catecholamines at presyncope which may limit compensatory elevations in cardiac contractility, heart rate or peripheral vasoconstriction (Convertino, 1998).

A gender comparison of orthostatic tolerance may be further complicated by potential effects of menstrual function. One hypothesis is that estrogens reduce vascular tone (Altura, 1975; von Eiff et al., 1971) which could result in greater peripheral blood flow or in less effective vasoconstrictor responses during ovulatory and/or luteal phases of the menstrual cycle (Hassan et al., 1990). Presumably this greater peripheral vasodilation could facilitate lower orthostatic tolerance. Although this hypothesis has not been critically evaluated using well-controlled orthostatic tolerance testing, investigators who have examined the cardiovascular responses to subtolerance levels of LBNP have reported no significant effect of menstrual phase (Frey et al., 1986; Rahman et al., 1991).

Another difficulty in comparing male and female responses to orthostasis is that each gender may use different compensatory mechanisms to maintain blood pressure. Women generally have lower resting blood pressures, higher cutaneous blood flow and respond to orthostasis to a greater extent by increasing heart rate than men (Frey et al., 1986; Vernikos et al., 1993). On the other hand, men generally have higher vasoconstrictor tone, increased central and total blood volume, and respond to orthostasis to a greater extent by increasing vasoconstrictor tone with an attenuated heart-rate response than do women (Montgomery et al., 1977). If women tend to be heart-rate responders, and if the change in heart rate to a given level of orthostatic stress is used to estimate orthostatic tolerance, then it may appear that women have lower orthostatic tolerance when only subtolerance responses are evaluated.

POTENTIAL MECHANISMS FOR ORTHOSTATIC AND HYPOTENSIVE INTOLERANCE AFTER BED REST

Orthostatic tolerance depends on appropriate interactions between the neural, hormonal, and endocrine systems. During prolonged BR these varying mechanisms may contribute to orthostatic intolerance depending on the length of BR exposure; this will further complicate the task of devising effective treatments. Discussed below are some of the possible mechanisms that contribute to orthostatic and hypotensive intolerance during BR.

Body Fluid Losses

One early response to even short BR is a loss of body water. Presumably the cephalic shift of fluids into the thoracic region stimulates atrial receptors resulting in peripheral vasodilation, increased renal perfusion, and increased urine loss (Gauer and Henry, 1963). However, Gilmore and Zucker (1978) have questioned the importance of this "Henry–Gauer reflex" for upright primates such as man. Norsk (1996) suggests that the fluid loss at the onset of BR is caused instead by changes in arterial baroreflex function. The diuresis during the first several hours of BR may be accompanied by reduced voluntary fluid intake thereby also contributing to the early negative fluid balance (Greenleaf, 1989).

This negative fluid balance results in an ultimate loss of plasma volume. Upon abruptly assuming the horizontal or head-down position there is an initial 6–7% expansion of plasma volume for about 1–2 hr followed immediately by a reduction after about 4 hr (Greenleaf, 1989). Thereafter, plasma volume decreases by about

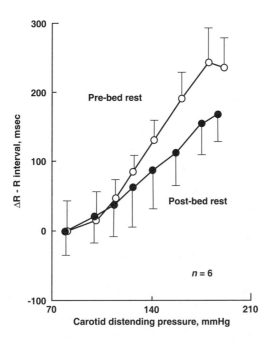

Figure 9.1   Change in the carotid sinus cardiac baroreflex after BR. Change in heart-rate, expressed in terms of R–R interval, is plotted against the change in carotid distending pressure induced with a neck chamber. Data are the responses of six subjects before and after 10 days of BR. (From Eckberg and Fritsch, 1991, with permission.)

20% until a new lower steady state is approached after about 30 days (Greenleaf et al., 1977). During short-term (<1 week) BR, the decrease in orthostatic response is proportional to the hypovolemia, and restoration of plasma volume improves orthostatic function (Gaffney et al., 1985; Hyatt and West, 1977).

With increasing duration of BR (> 1 week), the simple restoration of body fluids becomes progressively less effective for improving orthostatic responses. Following 14 days of BR, rehydration with a hypertonic salt solution improved acceleration tolerance to +2.1G_z in eight men (Greenleaf et al., 1973); but following 30 days of BR, performance of isotonic exercise training twice daily during BR maintained plasma volume but did not improve tilt-tolerance in seven men (Greenleaf et al., 1989).

Carotid-Cardiac Baroreceptor Function

When arterial blood pressure falls suddenly, carotid sinus and aortic arch baroreceptors are stimulated to increase heart rate and initiate peripheral vasoconstriction. The heart-rate response of the carotid baroreflex is characterized by a sigmoid-shaped curve; the slope and range of the curve are indicators of the ability of this reflex to compensate for a drop in blood pressure (Figure 9.1). After 10–12 days of BR this baroreflex curve is altered, showing a reduced maximal slope and a reduced range of blood pressure response (Convertino, 1990; Convertino et al., 1990; Eckberg and Fritsch, 1991). Subjects who had the greatest shift in baroreflex response also experienced the greatest impairment in post-BR orthostatic tolerance (Convertino, 1990; Convertino et al., 1990). The importance of this change in carotid cardiac baroreflex response on orthostatic tolerance may depend on the length of the BR and thus on the status of other cardio-acceleratory responses; for example the aortic baroreflex (Crandall et al., 1994), vestibular responses (Convertino et al., 1997), sympathetic/vagal balance, or the cardiac response to circulating catecholamines.

Autonomic Function

Changes in autonomic function could contribute to the development of orthostatic intolerance through several levels of action. Altered central autonomic balance, decreased neurotransmitter synthesis or release, and/or an altered end-organ sensitivity to adrenergic substances may all occur with inactivity or bed rest and result in inadequate cardiac or blood pressure compensatory responses.

Continuous beat-to-beat monitoring of the heart rate and blood pressure is often used as a simple non-invasive method of assessing the status of the autonomic nervous system. Heart-rate time-domain analyses express the data as a spectrum of heart-rate frequencies; the high-frequency domain (0.15 to 0.50 Hz) is used to characterize parasympathetic activity, and the low-frequency domain (0.0 to 0.15 Hz) characterizes sympathetic activity (Figure 9.2). A decreased ratio of high/low frequency domains and reduction in the total heart-rate variability, as reflected by the total spectrum, is clinically associated with greater orthostatic intolerance (Hughson et al., 1994).

During BR there are considerable decreases in the heart-rate and blood-pressure excursions normally associated with changes in posture and activity. Over time these attenuated excursions may result in resetting of the overall autonomic balance. For example, after 4 days of BR, Sigaudo et al. (1996) found a significant decrease in the high-frequency domain (parasympathetic activity) without change in the total or low-frequency domains. A similar decrease in parasympathetic domain, without change in sympathetic, was reported after 15 days of BR (Crandall et al., 1994b). However, after 20 hr (Patwardhan et al., 1995), 28 days (Hughson et al., 1994), and 42 days (Traon et al., 1998) of BR, decreases in the total and parasympathetic domain have been reported. This overall shift towards reduced parasympathetic and increased sympathetic domains (decreased high/low frequency ratio) most likely contribute to an exaggerated heart rate and blood pressure response to an orthostatic stress, such as tilt following BR.

The sustained decrease in sympathetic stimulation during BR, related to inactivity and reduced postural reflexes, results in a hypoadrenergic state. An indirect indicator of this state is a reduction in circulating and excreted norepinephrine levels. Convertino et al. (1998) reported a 40% reduction in total circulating NE after

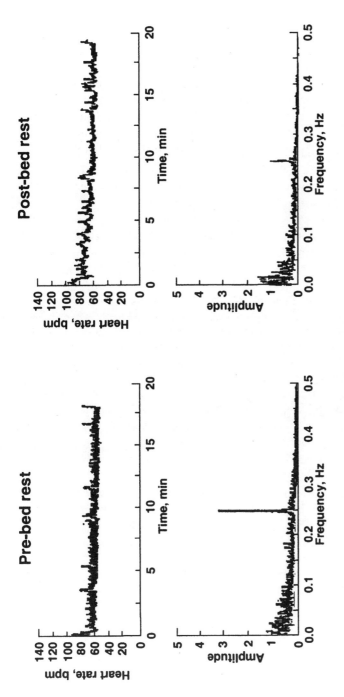

Figure 9.2 Heart-rate time series and spectra from a representative healthy adult female before and after 9 days of BR. There is a prominent, vagally mediated high-frequency peak pre-BR associated with metronomic breathing at 0.25 Hz. After bed rest there is an attenuation of this peak. (From Goldberger and Rigney, 1991, with permission.)

2 weeks of BR. A prolonged hypoadrenergic exposure has been postulated to result in either a decreased ability to secrete vasoconstrictor neurotransmitters or a down-regulation of alpha-adrenergic receptors. In the same study by Convertino et al. (1998), in which baseline NE levels were suppressed, NE release in response to a cold-pressor test was abolished after 14 and 27 days of BR. However, the vascular response to NE infusion was not altered, suggesting that the impairment in adrenergic function during BR was due to an inability to synthesize or release NE, and not to a down-regulation of the alpha-adrenergic receptors. Further data supporting impaired neural release and lack of change in vascular receptors was provided by Chobanian et al. (1974). They studied alpha-adrenergic function in six healthy men after 2–3 weeks of BR by measuring changes in mean arterial pressure following infusions of phenylephrine and angiotensin II. The infused doses of each drug necessary to produce a given increase in forearm vascular resistance and venous tone were not altered, suggesting no change in end-organ sensitivity. Similar negative findings of altered blood pressure responses to phenylephrine infusion after 14 days of BR were reported by Convertino et al. (1997), although these authors did find an attenuated response to angiotensin II infusion. Schmid et al. (1971) reported that the vasoconstrictor and venoconstrictor responses to tyramine infusion were attenuated after 12 days of BR, which would suggest decreased synthesis or storage of NE in pre-junctional nerve endings. Thus, the majority of data support a decreased release of NE from nerve endings after BR. A decreased release of NE in response to orthostatic simulus and/or decreased sensitivity of angiotension II receptors thus may contribute to possible impaired arterial vasoconstrictor or venoconstrictor responses to orthostasis after a prolonged period of BR.

An up-regulation of beta-adrenergic receptor function could result in increased heart rate and contractility, arterial venous dilation, and possibly impaired ability to vasoconstrict. Another possible mechanism for the impaired cardiovascular responses after bed rest might be an increased beta-adrenergic sensitivity. Evidence to support this theory includes potentiated heart rate and leg vasodilatory responses to graded iso-proterenol infusion following 14 days of BR as shown by Convertino et al. (1997). Earlier reports of an enhanced beta-adrenergic function during bed rest include additional isoproterenol infusion data from Melada et al. (1975) and a limited improvement in post-BR orthhostatic responses after beta-adrenergic blockade (Melada et al., 1975; Sandler et al., 1985).

Skeletal Muscle Tone

After only 20 hr of 5° head-down tilt, the supine resting stroke volume (SV) of five men was slightly smaller and the fall in SV in response to lower body negative pressure (LBNP) was much greater than before tilt (Gaffney et al., 1985). The smaller supine SV was most likely related to an 8% reduction in blood volume. However, the greater fall in SV during LBNP could be a result of an inadequate cardiac response (discussed below) or of a greater pooling of blood in the lower body. Some investigators (Convertino et al., 1989a,b; Louisy et al., 1990) have

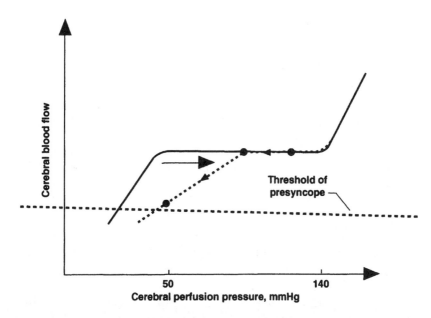

Figure 9.3 A possible shift in the cerebral autoregulation curve following BR. A dynamic rightward shift of the autoregulation curve means that a lower level of cerebral blood flow (CBF) will be attained at higher cerebral perfusion pressures (CPP) following BR. (Adapted from Bondar et al. (1995).)

suggested that the decrease in orthostatic tolerance after BR may result from a greater pooling of blood in the lower body, which may occur because of either an absolute loss of muscle mass in the leg muscles surrounding the veins or because of a generalized loss of skeletal muscle tone. Luft et al. (1976) reported a significant positive correlation between the degree of leg pooling during LBNP and orthostatic intolerance; and Convertino et al. (1988) have reported a significant negative correlation between the amount of muscle mass in the lower leg and leg distensibility. However, after accounting for the decrease in leg diameter that occurs during BR and that associated with fluid shifts and muscle atrophy, others did not report an increase in leg compliance during LBNP following 13 days of BR despite marked hypotensive intolerance in the subjects (Melchior and Fortney, 1993). Thus, loss of leg muscle tone and muscle mass may contribute to the decline in orthostatic-hypotensive tolerance, but this loss may become prominent only after the first couple of weeks of BR.

Cerebral Autoregulation

There is a transient increase in upper-body perfusion and cerebral blood flow that most likely contributes to the initial symptoms of headache and head fullness during the first few days of BR (Guell et al., 1982; Kawai et al., 1993). It is reasonable to expect, after prolonged exposure to the horizontal or head-down body position, that the adaptation to this redistribution of blood flow toward the head together with the reduced variations in cerebral perfusion owing to postural change, might affect cerebral autoregulation. Normally, cerebral blood flow is tightly controlled to maintain constant perfusion over a wide range (50–140 mmHg) of arterial blood pressure. With constant and prolonged exposure to an elevated pressure, it is possible that this autoregulation curve might be shifted to the right toward a constant perfusion at higher levels of arterial pressure (Figure 9.3). Such a shift, however, may result in an attenuated ability to maintain cerebral perfusion in response to a falling arterial pressure as suggested by an earlier and greater fall in cerebral blood flow during LBNP in 12 subjects after 2 weeks of BR (Zhang et al., 1997).

Venous Compliance

Including the liver and spleen, approximately 70% of the circulating blood volume resides in the venous system. Abnormalities in venous "tone" are considered the predominant non-cardiac mechanism for reduced tolerance in patients with orthostatic hypotension (Streeten and Scullard, 1996). In the upright body position the lower body veins are exposed to an hydrostatic pressure, thereby activating a local sympathetic response to increase smooth-muscle constriction to prevent blood pooling. Venous pooling is virtually eliminated in the lower limbs during BR, thus potentially compromising this local smooth-muscle response. Venous tone is also maintained during standing by neurally mediated baroreflex action and in response to circulating vasoactive substances.

Loss of venous tone has been suggested as a prominent contributing mechanism to post-BR orthostatic intolerance (Blamick et al., 1988; Convertino et al., 1989a,b; Convertino, 1990; Louisy et al., 1990; Menninger et al., 1969). Although most authors have located this pooling effect in the veins of the legs, a more important site for sequestering blood may be the abdomen. During exposure to –50 mmHg LBNP before 120 days of BR, splanchnic blood volume (estimated by radioisotope imaging) decreased by 3%, indicating a functioning venoconstrictor reflex response; following BR, the splanchnic blood volume increased instead of decreasing during LBNP (Savilov et al., 1990).

Cardiac Compliance

Until recently it was assumed that the cardiac function was not impaired by BR deconditioning. Heart size (estimated by echocardiography) initially increased during the first 6 hr of BR and then returned to the pre-BR value after 24 hr (Blomqvist et al., 1980). After 10 days of BR the supine left ventricular end diastolic volume was reduced by 16% (Hung et al., 1983) which was attributed to the ongoing changes in blood redistribution and volume. Cardiac contractility was maintained both at rest (Hung et al., 1983; Blomqvist et al., 1980) and during exercise (Hung et al., 1983) following BR.

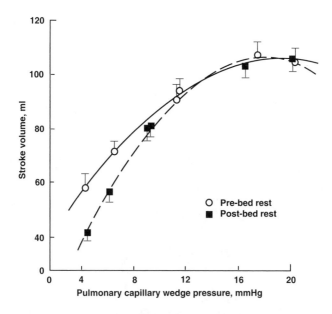

Figure 9.4 Change in the Starling curve relating cardiac filling (as estimated by the pulmo-nary wedge pressure (PWC) and stroke volume (measured by echocardiography) before and after 2 weeks of BR. This curve was created by reducing cardiac filling by application of –15 and –30 mmHg lower body negative pressure (the 2 lowest points) and by increasing cardiac filling by saline infusion of 15 and 30 mL/kg (the 2 highest points). The two middle points represent the baseline values before LBNP or saline infusion. (From Levine et al., 1997, with permission.)

More recently, however, Levine et al. (1997) reported decreases in cardiac mass and mechanics after only 2 weeks of BR and proposed that these cardiac changes contributed to the 24% reduction in LBNP tolerance in their 12 subjects. A surprising finding was that cardiac mass appeared to decrease by 5% ($P < 0.10$) during BR, which was consistent with cardiac atrophy. This decrease in cardiac mass, coupled with a change in the pressure-volume relationship of the heart, suggested decreased chamber distensibility which led to a steeper Starling relationship (Figure 9.4). Thus, after BR there appears to be not only reduced resting SV, but also a more precipitous fall in SV in response to any given drop in cardiac filling. Thus, changes in cardiac function may be an important contributor to orthostatic intolerance after only 2 weeks of BR.

COUNTERMEASURES TO PREVENT ORTHOSTATIC-HYPOTENSIVE INTOLERANCE DURING BED REST

With so many factors contributing to BR-induced orthostatic-hypotensive intoler-ance, it is not surprising that no single treatment or countermeasure has proved

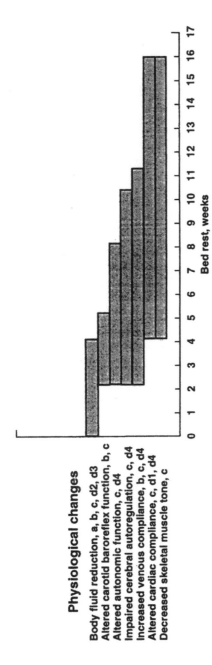

Figure 9.5 Summary of physiological changes during BR that may contribute to orthostatic-hypotensive intolerance and potential treatments.

effective. For example, fluid loading may be appropriate after 1 to 2 days, but it offers little benefit after a few weeks of BR. Data in Figure 9.5 illustrate the time-course for onset of some possible mechanisms for orthostatic intolerance during prolonged (120-day) BR. These results were compiled from numerous data in the literature that utilized varying BR models; for example, from horizontal to varying angles of HDT, and with various procedures for orthostatic-hypotensive testing. Potential treatments at these various times are also indicated.

Fluid/Salt Ingestion

Since fluid loss and reduction in plasma volume (PV) contribute to orthostatic into-lerance (Blomqvist et al., 1980) and may be a primary problem after short decondi-tioning exposures, a simple treatment would be to restore body fluids through oral hydration or infusion. This, however, becomes quite difficult if fluid restoration is started while the subject is supine. Without a hydrostatic gradient, additional hydr-ation is sensed by the body as an over-expansion of blood volume and it provokes a marked diuresis without sustained expansion of the plasma volume (Frey et al., 1991).

Another approach may be to increase salt intake acutely within hours of the end of BR. There is, however, a very tight balance between adding too little or too much salt to the rehydration solution. Too much salt (3% solution) stimulates reflexes to excrete the excess salt, whereas too little salt (0.45% solution) also triggers reflexes to normalize plasma osmolality by excreting the excess water (Fortney et al., 1994). In addition, the sodium content of the rehydration solution appears to be more important than the total osmolality (Greenleaf et al., 1998a; Greenleaf et al., 1998b). The most effective acute fluid loading treatment near the end of the BR may be an isotonic or only slightly hypertonic (1.1%) salt solution consisting of 157 mEq·L^{-1} Na, and an osmolality of 270 mOsm·kg^{-1} water (Greenleaf, 1998b). However, adding sugar or other osmotic substances to increase palatability of the solution may provoke a diuresis. A more palatable solution tested was isotonic bouillon (Frey et al., 1991; Fortney et al., 1994).

Maintenance of PV during 30 days of BR by chronic administration of either a higher (10 g/day) or lower (1 g/day) dietary salt intake, was compared to that during a normal diet of 4 g/day. Both the high- and low-salt diets resulted in a smaller PV compared with the normal diet by the end of 21 days of BR. The high-salt diet initially expanded PV, but induced decreased aldosterone and anti-diuretic hormone concentrations and increased atrial natriuretic factor levels which subsequently reduced PV (Williams et al., 1999).

Intermittent Tilt/LBNP

It is not clear that continuous BR is necessary to induce orthostatic intolerance. Vernikos et al. (1996) allowed subjects to stand or walk for either 2 or 4 hr each day during a 4-day, 6° head-down BR period. Orthostatic tolerance was assessed by time and hemodynamic responses to 30 min of 60° HUT. Although 2 hr of quiet standing only partially prevented orthostatic intolerance, 4 hr completely prevented it. Walking at a rate of 3 mi·hr^{-1} for 4 hr each day provided no additional benefit over standing. Therefore, only 4 hr each day of either real or simulated hydrostatic gradients may be sufficient to reverse BR-induced orthostatic intolerance.

Lower body negative pressure can simulate some effects of gravity by inducing fluid shifts from the upper to the lower body (Wolthuis et al., 1974). Exposure to LBNP may be expected to counteract many of the proposed mechanisms that contribute to hypotensive intolerance; for example, by stimulating arterial and cardiopulmonary baroreflexes, by provoking release of hormones that restore body fluids, or by stimulating leg vascular smooth muscle. Hyatt and West (1977) have shown that a 4-hr exposure to a mild level of LBNP (–30 mmHg) improved PV and orthostatic responses following 7 days of BR, and it was even more effective when the subjects ingested 1 liter of an isotonic saline solution (bouillon) during the LBNP treatment. On the other hand, 2 hr of LBNP plus similar fluid ingestion was not sufficient to maintain orthostatic tolerance during 13 days of BR (Fortney et al., 1992). Therefore, LBNP, like standing, may require at least a 4-hr daily treatment to be effective.

Exercise Training

Exercise training during BR would be expected to affect many of the potential mechanisms influencing orthostatic intolerance; for example, 1 hr of supine isotonic exercise daily during 30 days of 6° HDT BR maintained PV at control levels (Greenleaf et al., 1992). Exercise training also increases the sensitivity of the carotid cardiac baroreflex (Halliwill et al., 1996; Convertino, 1990) and would be expected to increase skeletal muscle tone, stimulate splanchnic vasoconstriction, increase cardiac contractility, increase cerebral blood flow (Thomas et al., 1989), and increase sympathetic tone. Therefore, it is surprising that use of exercise training to restore orthostatic function during BR has produced mostly negative results (Birkhead et al., 1966; Greenleaf et al., 1989); with a few exceptions when the training was combined with a simultaneous orthostatic stressor—either upright exercise (Birkhead et al., 1964; Sullivan et al., 1985) or exercise during LBNP (Watenpaugh et al., 1994). Whether exercise training can reduce the required time of exposure to an upright or simulated upright posture to maintain orthostatic or hypotensive tolerance is unclear. One possible effect of the training is to redistribute blood flow away from the central volume into exercising muscles, which may increase the effectiveness of a tilt or LBNP countermeasure.

A single bout of maximal exercise has been shown to reduce the incidence of orthostatic intolerance following 16 days of BR (Engelke et al., 1996). Maximal exercise following such a relatively short BR exposure is thought to restore plasma volume, improve vasoconstrictor and cardiac baroreceptor sensitivity and possibly prevent attenuation of maximal NE secretion. A single bout of maximal arm exercise was shown to eliminate orthostatic hypotension in paraplegic patients (Engelke et al., 1994).

Pharmacological Treatments

Various pharmacological treatments tested after BR have met with only partial success in preventing orthostatic intolerance. The major difficulty in using drugs is that treatment of a condition with multiple causative factors would require a cocktail of drugs, all with potentially undesirable side effects.

Dobutamine is a synthetic catecholamine that stimulates alpha- and beta-adrenergic receptors that induce cardiovascular responses similar to those that occur during exercise. Results of dobutamine infusion have not demonstrated significant improvement in orthostatic function during hind-limb suspension in rats (Tipton and Sebastian, 1997) or during BR in humans (Sullivan et al., 1985).

Other drugs that offer some protection against orthostatic intolerance in hospitalized patients that might improve orthostatic intolerance in healthy people include the fluorohydrocorticoids (Bohnn et al., 1970; Vernikos et al., 1991) or antidiuretic hormone analogues (Kochar, 1985) which could restore body fluids and provide some improvement during short-duration BR. Alpha-adrenergic angonists such as midodrine (Low et al., 1997) and ergotamine (Biaggioni et al., 1990) might enhance vascular constriction and offer some protection especially during longer (>2 wk) BR. Similarly beta-adrenergic blockers such as propranolol have been suggested for maintenance of vascular tone following BR (Sandler et al., 1985).

PRACTICAL CONSIDERATIONS FOR ORTHOSTATIC INTOLERANCE AND THE BED-RESTED PATIENT

Orthostatic intolerance can be a problem even for healthy individuals after a few hours of BR. Upon reambulation, the longer the BR period the longer the recovery of blood pressure control. Potentially complicating effects from illness or medication may greatly increase the susceptibility to orthostatic intolerance. This may be of special concern for older patients with weakened bones, atrophied muscles, or impaired postural control. Such patients should be moved to an upright or semi-upright posture for at least 4 hr each day and encouraged to move their legs, especially when in the upright position. They should be assisted during the first few hours and even the first few days after arising and warned against the hazards of exposure to a hot shower or a hot environment which can increase susceptibility to fainting. Extra fluid and salt in their diet during the days before reambulation, and extra fluid ingestion for the first few days after arising, may accelerate their recovery. Vasoconstrictor and especially venoconstrictor counter-measures may be required for patients who do not recover rapidly upon reambulation. Mechanical supports such as elastic stockings or abdominal compression could be used in preference to pharmacological treatment.

REFERENCES

Altura, B. M. (1975) Sex and oestrogens and responsiveness of terminal arterioles to neurohypophyseal hormones and catecholamines. *J. Pharmacol. Exp. Ther.* **193**: 403–412.

Biaggioni, I., Zygmunt, D., Haile, V., and Robertson, D. (1990) Pressor effect of inhaled ergotamine in orthostatic hypotension. *Am. J. Cardiol.* **65**: 8–92.

Birkhead, N. C., Blizzard, J. J., Daly, J. W., Haupt, G. J., Issekutz, B., Jr., Myers, R. N., and Rodahl, K. (1964) Cardiodynamic and metabolic effects of prolonged bed rest with daily recumbent or sitting exercise and with sitting inactivity. Aerospace Medical Research Laboratories, Wright-Patterson Air Force Base, Ohio, AMRL-TDR-64-61, 28 pp.

Birkhead, N. C., Blizzard, J. J., Issekutz, B., and Rodahl, K. (1966) Effect of exercise, standing, negative trunk and positive skeletal pressure on bed-rest-induced orthostasis and hypercalciuria. Aerospace Medical Research Laboratories, Wright-Patterson Air Force Base, Ohio, AMRL-TR-66-6, 29 pp.

Blamick, C. A., Goldwater, D. J., and Convertino, V. A. (1988) Leg vascular responsiveness during acute orthostasis following simulated weightlessness. *Aviat. Space Environ. Med.* **59**: 40–43.

Blomqvist, C. G., Nixon, J. V., Johnson, R. L., and Mitchell, J. H. (1980) Early cardiovascular adaptation to zero gravity simulated by head-down tilt. *Acta Astronautica* **7**: 543–553.

Bohnn, B. J., Hyatt, K. H., Kamenetsky, L. G., Calder, B. E., and Smith, W. M. (1970) Prevention of bed-rest-induced orthostatism by 9-alpha-fluorohydrocortisone. *Aerospace Med.* **41**: 495–499.

Bondar, R. L., Kassam, M. S., Stein, F., Dunphy, P. T., Fortney, S., and Riedesel, M. L. (1995) Simultaneous cerebrovascular and cardiovascular responses during presyncope. *Stroke* **26**: 1794–1800.

Butler, G. C., Xing, H. C., Northey, D. R., and Hughson, R. L. (1991) Reduced orthostatic tolerance following 4 h head-down tilt. *Eur. J. Appl. Physiol.* **62**: 26–30.

Chobanian, A. V., Lille, R. D., Tercyak, A., and Blevins, P. (1974) The metabolic and hemodynamic effects of prolonged bed rest in normal subjects. *Circulation* **49**: 551–559.

Convertino, V. A. (1990) Carotid-cardiac baroreflex: relation with orthostatic hypotension following simulated microgravity and implications for development of countermeasures. *Acta Astronautica* **23**: 9–17.

Convertino, V. A. (1998) Gender differences in autonomic functions associated with blood pressure regulation. *Am. J. Physiol.* **275** *(Regulatory Integrative Comp. Physiol.* **44**): R1909–R1920.

Convertino, V. A., Adams, W. C., Shea, J. D., Thompson, C. A., and Hoffler, G. W. (1991) Impairment of carotid-cardiac vagal baroreflex in wheelchair-dependent quadriplegics. *Am. J. Physiol. Regulatory Integrative Comp. Physiol.* **260**: R576–R580.

Convertino, V. A., Doerr, D. F., Eckberg, D. L., Fritsch, J. M., and Vernikos-Danellis, J. (1990) Head-down bed rest impairs vagal baroreflex responses and provokes orthostatic hypotension. *J. Appl. Physiol.* **68**: 1458–1464.

Convertino, V. A., Doerr, D. F., Flores, J. F., Hoffler, G. W., and Buchanan, P. (1988) Leg size and muscle functions associated with leg compliance. *J. Appl. Physiol.* **64**: 1017–1021.

Convertino, V. A., Doerr, D. F., Mathes, K. L., Stein, S. L., and Buchanan, P. (1989a) Changes in volume, muscle compartment, and compliance of the lower extremeties in man following 30 days of exposure to simulated microgravity. *Aviat. Space Environ. Med.* **60**: 653–658.

Convertino, V. A., Doerr, D. F., and Stein, S. L. (1989b) Changes in size and compliance of the calf after 30 days of simulated microgravity. *J. Appl. Physiol.* **66**: 1509–1512.

Convertino, V. A., Ludwig, D. A., Gray, B. D., and Vernikos, J. (1998) Effects of exposure to simulated microgravity on neuronal catecholamine release and blood pressure responses to norepinephrine and angiotensin. *Clin. Auton. Res.* **8**: 101–110.

Convertino, V. A., Polet, J. L., Engelke, K. A., Hoffler, G. W., Lane, L. D., and Blomqvist, C. G. (1997) Evidence for increased β-adrenergic responsiveness induced by 14 days of simulated microgravity in humans. *Am. J. Physiol.* **273** *(Regulatory Integrative Comp. Physiol.* **42**): R93–R99.

Convertino, V. A., Previc, F. H., Ludwig, D. A., and Engelken, E. J. (1997) Effects of vestibular and oculomotor simulation on responsiveness of the carotid-cardiac baroreflex. *Am. J. Physiol. Regulatory Integrative Comp. Physiol.* **42**: R615–R622.

Crandall, C. G., Engelke, K. A., Convertino, V. A., and Raven, P. B. (1994a) Aortic baroreflex control of heart rate after 15 days of simulated microgravity exposure. *J. Appl. Physiol.* **77**: 2134–2139.

Crandall, C. G., Engelke, K. A., Pawelczyk, J. A., Raven, P. B., and Convertino, V. A. (1994b) Power spectral and time based analysis of heart rate variability following 15 days head-down bed rest. *Aviat. Space Environ. Med.* **65**: 1105–1109.

Denq, J.-C., Opfer-Gehrking, T. L., Giuliani, M., Felten, J., Convertino, V. A., and Low, P. A. (1997) Efficacy of compression of different capacitance beds in the amelioration of orthostatic hypotension. *Clin. Auton. Res.* **7**: 321–326.

Eckberg, D. L., and Fritsch, J. M. (1991) Human autonomic responses to actual and simulated weightlessness. *J. Clin. Pharmacol.* **31**: 951–955.

Engelke, K. A., Doerr, D. F., and Convertino, V. A. (1996) Application of acute maximal exercise to protect orthostatic tolerance after simulated microgravity. *Am. J. Physiol.* **271** *(Regulatory Integrative Comp. Physiol.* **40**): R837–R847.

Engelke, K. A., Shea, J. D., Doerr, D. F., and Convertino, V. A. (1994) Autonomic functions and orthostatic responses 24 h after acute intense exercise in paraplegic subjects. *Am. J. Physiol.* **266** *(Regulatory Integrative Comp. Physiol.* **35**:) R1189–R1196.

Fortney, S. M., Schneider, V. S., and Greenleaf, J. E. (1996) The physiology of bed rest. In *Handbook of Physiology*: Section 4: *Environmental Physiology*, edited by M. J. Fregly and C. M. Blatteis, Oxford University Press: New York, Vol. 2, Chap. 39, pp. 889–939.

Fortney, S. M., Steinmann, L., Dussack, L., Wood, M., Cintron, N., and Whitson, P. (1992) Investigations of the mechanisms by which lower body negative pressure (LBNP) improves orthostatic responses. 43rd Congress of the International Astronautical Federation, 1992, IAP/IAA-92-0263, Washington, DC.

Fortney, S. M., Steinmann, L., Young, J. A., Hoskin, C. N., and Barrows, L. H. (1994) Fluid-loading solutions and plasma volume: astro-ade and salt tablets with water. Houston, TX, NASA TP-3456, 25 pp.

Frey, M. A. B., and Hoffler, G. W. (1988) Association of sex and age with responses to lower-body negative pressure. *J. Appl. Physiol.* **65**: 1752–1756.

Frey, M. A. B., Mathes, K. L., and Hoffler, G. W. (1986) Cardiovascular responses of women to lower body negative pressure. *Aviat. Space Environ. Med.* **57**: 531–538.

Frey, M. A. B., Riddle, J., Charles, J. B., and Bungo, M. W. (1991) Blood and urine responses to ingesting fluids of various salt and glucose concentrations. *J. Clin. Pharmacol.* **31**: 8880–8887.

Gaffney, F. A., Nixon, J. V., Erling, M. D., Karlsson, S., Campbell, W., Dowdey, A. B. C., and Blomqvist, C. G. (1985) Cardiovascular deconditioning produced by 20 hours of bed rest with head-down tilt (−5°) in middle-aged healthy men. *Am. J. Cardiol.* **56**: 634–638.

Gauer, O. H., and Henry, J. P. (1963) Circulatory basis of fluid volume control. *Physiol. Rev.* **43**: 423–481.

Gilmore, J. P., and Zucker, I. H. (1978) Failure of left atrial distention to alter renal function in the nonhuman primate. *Circ. Res.* **42**: 267–270.

Goldberger, A. L., and Rigney, D. R. (1991) Cardiovascular dynamics during space sickness and deconditioning. In *Proceedings of the First Joint NASA Cardiopulmonary Workshop*, edited by S. Fortney and A. R. Hargens, NASA CR-10068, pp. 155–163.

Gotshall, R. W. (2000) Gender differences in tolerance to lower body negative pressure. *Aviat. Space Environ. Med.* **71**: 1104–1110.

Greenleaf, J. E. (1989) Hormonal regulation of fluid and electrolytes during prolonged bed-rest: implications for microgravity. In *Hormonal Regulation of Fluid and Electrolytes*, edited by J. R. Claybaugh and C. E. Wade, Plenum Publishing Corp.: New York, pp. 215–232.

Greenleaf, J. E., Bernauer, E. M., Young, H. L., Morse, J. T., Staley, R. W., Juhos, L. T., and Van Beaumont, W. (1977) Fluid and electrolyte shifts during bed rest with isometric and isotonic exercise. *J. Appl. Physiol.* **42**: 59–66.

Greenleaf, J. E., Jackson, C. G. R., Geelen, G., Keil, L. C., Hinghofer-Szalkay, H., and Whittam, J. H. (1998a) Plasma volume expansion with oral fluids in hypohydrated men at rest and during exercise. *Aviat. Space Environ. Med.* **69**: 837–844.

Greenleaf, J. E., Looft-Wilson, R., Wisherd, J. L., Jackson, C. G. R., Fung, P. P., Ertl, A. C., Barnes, P. R., Jensen, C. D., and Whittam, J. H. (1998b) Hypervolemia in men from fluid ingestion at rest and during exercise. *Aviat. Space Environ. Med.* **69**: 374–386.

Greenleaf, J. E., Van Beaumont, W., Bernauer, E. M., Haines, R. F., Sandler, H., Staley, R.W., Young, H. L., and Yusken, J. W. (1973) Effects of rehydration on +Gz tolerance after 14-days bed rest. *Aerospace Med.* **44**: 715–722.

Greenleaf, J. E., Vernikos, J., Wade, C. E., and Barnes, P. R. (1992) Effect of leg exercise training on vascular volumes during 30 days of 6° head-down bed rest. *J. Appl. Physiol.* **72**: 1887–1894.

Greenleaf, J. E., Wade, C. E., and Leftheriotis, G. (1989) Orthostatic responses following 30-day bed rest deconditioning with isotonic and isokinetic exercise training. *Aviat. Space Environ. Med.* **60**: 537–542.

Guell, A., Dupui, P. H., Barrere, M., Fanjaud, G., and Bes, A. (1982) Changes in the loco-regional cerebral blood flow (r.C.B.F.) during a simulation of weightlessness. *Acta Astronautica* **9**: 689–690.

Halliwill, J. R., Taylor, J. A., Hartwig, T. D., and Eckberg, D. L. (1996) Augmented baroreflex heart rate gain after moderate-intensity, dynamic exercise. *Am. J. Physiol. Regulatory Integrative Comp. Physiol.* **270**: R420–R426.

Harper, C. M., and Lyles, Y. M. (1988) Physiology and complications of bed rest. *J. Am. Geriatr. Soc.* **36**: 1047–1054.

Hassan, A. A. K., Carter, G., Tooke, J. E. (1990) Postural vasoconstriction during the normal menstrual cycle. *Clin. Sci.* **78**: 39–47.

Hordinsky, J. R., Gebhardt, U., Wegmann, H. M., and Schafer, G. (1981) Cardiovascular and biochemical response to simulated space flight entry. *Aviat. Space Environ. Med.* **52**: 16–18.

Hughson, R. L., Yamamoto, Y., Maillet, A., Fortrat, J. O., Traon, A. P., Butler, G. C., Guell, A., and Gharib, C. (1994) Altered autonomic regulation of cardiac function during head-up tilt after 28-day head-down bed rest with counter-measures. *Clin. Physiol.* **14**: 291–304.

Hung, H., Goldwater, D., Convertino, V. A., McKillop, J. H., Goris, M. L., and Debusk, R. F. (1983) Mechanisms for decreased exercise capacity after bed rest in normal middle-aged men. *Am. J. Cardiol.* **51**: 344–348.

Hyatt, K. H., and West, D. A. (1977) Reversal of bedrest-induced orthostatic intolerance by lower body negative pressure and saline. *Aviat. Space Environ. Med.* **48**: 120–124.

Kawai, Y., Murthy, G., Watenapaugh, D. E., Breit, G. A., Deroshia, C. W., and Hargens, A. R. (1993) Cerebral blood flow velocity in humans exposed to 24 h of head-down tilt. *J. Appl. Physiol.* **74**: 3046–3051.

Kochar, M. S. (1985) Hemodynamic effects of lysine-vasopressin in orthostatic hypotension. *Am. J. Kidney Dis.* **6**: 49–52.

Lamb, L. E., Johnson, R. L., Stevens, P. M., and Welch, B. E. (1964) Cardiovascular deconditioning from space cabin simulator confinement. *Aerospace Med.* **35**: 420–428.

Lathers, C. M., and Charles, J. B. (1993) Use of lower body negative pressure to counter symptoms of orthostatic intolerance in patients, bed rest subjects, and astronauts. *J. Clin. Pharmacol.* **33**:1071–1085.

Levine, B. D., Zuckerman, J. H., and Pawelczyk, J. A. (1997) Cardiac atrophy after bed-rest deconditioning: a non-neural mechanism for orthostatic intolerance. *Circulation* **96**: 517–525.

Lightfoot, J. T. and Tsintgiras, K. M. (1995) Quantification of tolerance to lower body negative pressure in a healthy population. *Med. Sci. Sports Exerc.* **27**: 697–706.

Louisy, F., Gaudin, C., Oppert, J. M., Guell, A., and Guezennec, C. Y. (1990) Haemodynamics of leg veins during a 30 days-6-degrees head-down bedrest with and without lower body negative pressure. *Eur. J. Appl. Physiol.* **61**: 349–355.

Low, P. A., Gilden, J. L., Freeman, R., Sheng, K. N., and McElligott, M. A. (1997) Efficacy of midodrine vs. placebo in neurogenic orthostatic hypotension: a randomized, double-blind multicenter study. Midodrine Study Group. *J.A.M.A.* **277**: 1046–1051.

Luft, U. C., Myhre, L. G., Loeppky, J. A., and Venters, M. D. (1976) A study of factors affecting tolerance to gravitational stress simulated by lower body negative pressure. Lovelace Foundation: Albuquerque, NM, 60 pp.

Melada, G. A., Goldman, R. H. , Luetscher, J. A., and Zager, P. G. (1975) Hemodynamics, renal function, plasma renin, and aldosterone in man after 5 to 14 days of bed-rest. *Aviat. Space Environ. Med.* **46**: 1049–1055.

Melchior, F. M., and Fortney, S. M. (1993) Orthostatic intolerance during a 13-day bed-rest does not result from increased leg compliance. *J. Appl. Physiol.* **74**: 286–292.

Menninger, R. P., Mains, R. C., Zechman, F. W., and Piemme, T. A. (1969) Effect of two weeks bed rest on venous pooling in the lower limbs. *Aerospace Med.* **40**: 1323–1326.

Montgomery, L. D., Kirk, P. J., Payne, P. A., Gerber, R. L., Newton, S. D., and Williams, B. A. (1977) Cardiovascular responses of men and women to lower body negative pressure. *Aviat. Space Environ. Med.* **48**: 138–145.

Norsk, P. (1996) Role of arginine vasopressin in the regulation of extracellular fluid volume. *Med. Sci. Sports Exerc.* **28**: *Suppl* 10: S36–S41.

Pannier, B. M., Lacolley, P. J., Gharib, C., London, G. M., Cuche, J. L., Duchier, J. L., Levy, B. I., and Safar, M. E. (1991) Twenty-four hours of bed rest with head-down tilt: venous and arteriolar changes in limbs. *Am. J. Physiol. Heart Circ. Physiol.* **260**: H1043–H1050.

Patwardhan, A. R., Evans, J. M., Berk, M., Grande, K. J., Charles, J. B., and Knapp, C. F. (1995) Spectral indices of cardiovascular adaptations to short-term simulated microgravity exposure. *Integr. Physiol. Behav. Sci.* **30**: 201–214.

Rahman, M. A., Goodhead, K., Medcalf, J. F., O'Connor, M., and Bennett, T. (1991) Haemodynamic responses to nonhypotensive central hypovolemia induced by lower body negative pressure in men and women. *Eur. J. Appl. Physiol.* **63**: 151–155.

Raven, P. B., Welch-O'Connor, R. M., and Shi, X. (1998) Cardiovascular function following reduced aerobic activity. *Med. Sci. Sports Exerc.* **30**: 1041–1052.

Sandler, H., Goldwater, D. J., Popp, R. L., Spaccavento, L., and Harrison, D. C. (1985) Beta blockade in the compensation for bed-rest cardiovascular deconditioning: physiological and pharmacologic observations. *Am. J. Cardiol.* **55**: 114D–119D.

Savilov, A. A., Lobachik, V. I., and Babin, A. M. (1990) Cardiovascular function of man exposed to LBNP tests. *Physiologist* **33**: S128–S132.

Schmid, P. G., McCally, M., Piemme, T. E., and Shaver, J. A. (1971) Effects of bed rest on forearm vascular responses to tyramine and norepinephrine. In *Hypogravic and Hypodynamic Environments*, edited by R. H. Murray and M. McCally, Washington, DC, NASA SP-269, pp. 211–223.

Shi, X., Squires, W. G., Williamson, J. W., Crandall, C. G., Chen, J. J., Krock, L. P., and Raven, P. B. (1992) Aerobic fitness: 1. Response of volume regulating hormones to head-down tilt. *Med. Sci. Sports Exerc.* **24**: 991–998.

Sigaudo, D., Fortrat, J. O., Maillet, A., Allevard, A. M., Traon, A. P. L., Hughson, R. L., Guell, A., Gharib, C., and Gauquelin, G. (1996) Comparison of a 40-day confinement and head-down tilt on endocrine response and cardiovascular variability in humans. *Eur. J. Appl. Physiol.* **73**: 28–37.

Streeten, D. H. P., and Scullard, T. F. (1996) Excessive gravitational blood pooling caused by impaired venous tone is the predominant non-cardiac mechanism of orthostatic intolerance. *Clin. Sci.* **90**: 277–285.

Sullivan, M. J., Binkley, F., Unvergerth, D. V., Ren, J. H., Boudoulas, H., Bashore, T. M., Merola, A. J., and Leier, C. V. (1985) Prevention of bed-rest-induced physical deconditioning by daily dobutamine infusions. *J. Clin. Invest.* **76**: 1632–1642.

Thomas, S. N., Schroeder, T., Secher, N. H., and Mitchell, J. H. (1989) Cerebral blood flow during submaximal and maximal dynamic exercise in humans. *J. Appl. Physiol.* **67**: 744–748.

Tipton, C. M., and Sebastian, L. A. (1997) Dobutamine as a countermeasure for reduced exercise performance of rats exposed to simulated microgravity. *J. Appl. Physiol.* **82**: 1607–1615.

Traon, A. P. L., Sigaudo, D., Vasseur, P., Maillet, A., Fortrat, J. O., Hughson, R. L., Gauquelin-Koch, G., and Gharib, C. (1998) Cardiovascular responses to orthostatic tests after a 42-day head-down bed-rest. *Eur. J. Appl. Physiol.* **77**: 50–59.

Vernikos, J., Dallman, M. F., Keil, L. C., O'Hare, D., and Convertino, V. A. (1993) Gender differences in endocrine responses to posture and 7 days of −6° head down bed-rest. *Am. J. Physiol. Endocrinol. Metab.* **265**: E153–E161.

Vernikos, J., Dallman, M. F., Van Loon, G., and Keil, L. C. (1991) Drug effects on orthostatic intolerance induced by bed-rest. *J. Clin. Pharmacol.* **31**: 974–984.

Vernikos, J., Ludwig, D. A., Ertl, A. C., Wade, C. E., Keil, L., and O'Hare, D. (1996) Effect of standing and walking on physiological changes induced by head-down bed rest: implications for spaceflight. *Aviat. Space Environ. Med.* **67**: 1069–1079.

Vogt, F. B. (1967) Tilt table and plasma volume changes with short term deconditioning experiments. *Aerospace Med.* **38**: 564–568.

Von Eiff, A. W., Plotz, E. J., Beck, K. J., and Czernik, A. (1971) The effect of estrogens and progesterones on blood pressure regulation of normotensive women. *Am. J. Obstet. Gynecol.* **109**: 887–892.

Watenpaugh, D. E., Fortney, S. M., Ballard, R. E., Lee, S. M. C., Bennett, B. S., Murthy, G., Kramer, G. C., and Hargens, A. R. (1994) Lower body negative pressure during bed-rest maintains orthostatic tolerance. *FASEB J.* **8**: A261.

White, D. D., Gotshall, R. W., and Tucker, A. (1996) Women have lower tolerance to lower body negative pressure than men. *J. Appl. Physiol.* **80**: 1138–1143.

Williams, W. J., Lee, S. M. C., Stuart, C. A., Whitson, P. A., and Schneider, S. M. (1999) Effect of bed-rest and dietary sodium on forearm blood flow (FBF) during lower body negative pressure (LBNP). *FASEB J.* **13**: A405.

Wolthuis, R. A., Bergman, S. A., and Nicogossian, A. E. (1974) Physiological effects of locally applied reduced pressure in man. *Physiol. Rev.* **54**: 566–595.

Zhang, R., Zuckerman, J. H., Pawelczyk, J. A., and Levine, B. D. (1997) Effects of head-down bed rest on cerebral hemodynamics during orthostatic stress. *J. Appl. Physiol.* **83**: 2139–2145.

CHAPTER 10

Thermoregulation during Deconditioning

Suzanne M. Schneider[1] and John E. Greenleaf[2]

[1]*Department of Physical Performance and Development, University of New Mexico, Albuquerque, New Mexico, USA*
[2]*Laboratory for Human Environmental Physiology, NASA, Ames Research Center, Moffett Field, California, USA*

> Man is the shuttle, to whose winding quest
> And passage through these looms
> God order'd motion, but ordain'd no rest.
>
> *Henry Vaughan*

INTRODUCTION

The importance of maintaining body temperature is well understood by both clinicians and lay persons. The normal, resting body core temperature (T_{co}) is about 37°C (98.6°F), and death often occurs when it falls below 27°C (80.6°F) or exceeds 42°C (107.6°F). Thus, for survival, the degree of overheating is more critical than that for overcooling. The lower limit of T_{co} for onset of heatstroke is usually only 41–42°C (105.8–107.6°F) (Shibolet et al., 1976), but classic heatstroke has occurred with T_{co} as low as 40.6°C (105.1°F) (Leithead and Lind, 1964).

Not only the absolute level of T_{co}, but also the rate of heat exchange is important in the onset of heat maladies. Unacclimated men resting in a hot, humid environment —42°C (107.6°F) and a relative humidity (rh) of 90%—can be near their limits of tolerance and consciousness with T_{co} of 38.5°C (101.3°F) (Convertino et al., 1980). However, during intense exercise, rectal temperatures (T_{re}) in the heatstroke range have occurred with no lasting adverse signs or symptoms. Robinson (1963) measured rectal temperatures of 40.0 and 41.1°C (104.0 and 105.9°F) in two runners after a 5-km race, and Pugh et al. (1967) observed temperatures of 41.1, 40.5, and

40.2°C (104.0, 104.9, and 104.4°F, respectively) in the first-, third-, and fourth-place finishers, respectively, of a marathon race. Under normal ambient conditions, heat exhaustion (caused by dehydration and excessive salt loss) and physical debilitation usually occur before the onset of heatstroke (which is often associated with cessation of sweating). When heat flow from the body is reduced, such as when astronauts work in an extra-vehicular-activity (EVA) suit at a rate such that heat removal is significantly less than heat production, skin temperature rises. This rise in skin temperature then results in a reduced core-to-skin temperature gradient, which causes T_{co} to rise. Under such conditions of attenuated heat dissipation, significant signs and symptoms of heat stress can occur at T_{co} as low as 38°C (100.4°F) (Smith, 1980; Tanaka et al., 1978). Thus, without knowledge of the situation in which the temperature is measured, it is clear that the absolute value of T_{co} per se cannot be used to determine the physiological states of workers or astronauts, or to predict when heat exhaustion or heatstroke are likely to occur.

Humans are uniquely prepared to defend their body thermoregulatory state, especially against increases in body temperature. They possess very effective and efficient sweating and vasodilatory reflexes which are activated as soon as T_{co} exceeds a threshold value; the threshold value varies depending on the state of hydration, fitness, heat acclimation, time of day, or (in females) the phase of the menstrual cycle.

Adverse changes in thermoregulation during spaceflight could significantly affect the comfort, performance, and even survival of crew members. In a normal environment, behavioral modifications can maintain body temperature under all but the most extreme conditions. However, during flight, the confinement and restricted resources limit astronauts' ability to alter environmental conditions or activity levels. When environmental control fails—such as during the recent Mir 19 mission when leaks in the cooling system sent cabin temperatures to 36°C (96.8°F) for several days; and during the Apollo 13 mission when the crew, returning from a failed Moon landing, was exposed to near freezing temperatures for several days—appropriate thermoregulatory responses become critical. Thermoregulation may also be compromised when crew members wear impermeable clothing such as the EVA suit or a launch and entry suit (LES), even though these garments contain liquid cooling systems. For example; if the cooling system malfunctions, if the crew must work harder than expected, or if they must disconnect from the cooling system as they might during an emergency landing, then heat loss would be attenuated and body temperatures could rise to lethal levels within minutes (Pandolf et al., 1995).

During long-duration space missions it is expected that crew members will exercise and this might help them maintain thermoregulatory capacity. On the other hand, it is probable that they will lose their heat acclimation status since many of them exercise in the heat and humidity of Houston, Texas. It is probable that crew members lose body fluids during spaceflight, but this is still an open question. When body fluid compartments were measured in seven crew members during the SLS-1 and SLS-2 Shuttle missions, *extracellular* fluid volume was reduced but the volume of total body water was unchanged from preflight levels. These surprising results suggest that there is a redistribution of body water from the extracellular to the cellular fluid compartment (Leach et al., 1996). Nonetheless, a reduction in extracellular volume would have a negative effect on thermoregulation in both hot (Sawka et al., 1992, Fortney et al., 1981) and cold (O'Brien et al., 1998) environments.

Other homeostatic changes associated with prolonged spaceflight may affect thermoregulation and thus crew performance or comfort. The normal 24-hr circadian change in body temperature is disrupted with exposure to the 90-min day/night cycles in orbital flight (Czeisler et al., 1991; Lhagwa, 1984). Lack of appropriate circadian temperature fluctuations may affect crew sleep, alertness, and cognitive function. In response, the crew frequently uses pharmacological aids to help them sleep and stay alert. However, the pharmokinetics of some drugs used in weightlessness may be impaired, thus resulting in a need for stronger dosages in space than are used on the ground (Putcha et al., 1999). And some of these drugs (e.g., sleeping medications, adrenergic stimulants) can interfere with normal thermoregulatory function.

The physical effects of weightlessness on heat loss responses have not been well investigated; however, convective heat loss is greatly compromised and evaporative heat loss may also be impaired (Leach et al., 1978). These effects on convection and evaporation can be minimized by increasing air flow and reducing ambient humidity. The specific environments that crew members may be expected to encounter are described below.

SPACEFLIGHT ENVIRONMENT

Intravehicular Activities: Shuttle, Mir, International Space Station

Beginning with Skylab flights in 1973 all American space vehicles for humans, as well as the Russian Mir and the International Space Station (ISS), have been designed to maintain an atmosphere similar to that on Earth. During long-duration spaceflights crew members are required to perform rather intense aerobic and resistive exercise as countermeasures in an effort to maintain in-flight health and to prepare them for a successful landing. Despite the almost daily exercise, however, all crew members have significant difficulty maintaining exercise and orthostatic capacities throughout long-duration flights.

Shuttle

The Shuttle environmental control system was designed to maintain ambient temperature between 18 and 27°C (64.4 and 80.6°F), relative humidity between 23 and 90%, and a variable air flow between 0.1 and 0.2 m·sec^{-1} (Waligora et al., 1994). The atmospheric environment in the Shuttle is maintained at 101.3 kPa (14.7 psi) with a gas composition of approximately 80% N_2, 20% O_2, with less than 0.5 % CO_2.

In-flight exercise training is required of all crew members on American flights that last longer than 10 days. The Shuttle flight exercise program requires at least 20 min of aerobic exercise every other day for the flight crew (pilot, copilot, and navigator) and every third day for mission and payload specialists. The exercise devices available on Shuttle flights have included a treadmill, a cycle ergometer, or a rower.

Mir

On the Russian Mir space station the atmospheric ranges are similar to the American guidelines: 19.9 to 22.5% O_2, 0.7 to 1.0% CO_2 with the balance N_2; ambient temperature is maintained between 18 and 28°C (64.4 and 82.4°F), the relative humidity between 30 and 70%, and the airflow between 0.05 and 0.2 m·sec^{-1} (Wieland, 1998).

During Mir missions, which typically last 3–4 months but some have lasted longer than a year, all crew members perform approximately 1–2 hr of exercise daily but the schedule varies depending on the stage of the mission. Late in the mission the exercise sessions increase in intensity, frequency, and duration. The Russian exercise countermeasure program consists of aerobic cycle or treadmill exercises interspersed with stretching and resistive exercises against bungi cord expanders. Exercise intensity is prescribed individually for the crew. Heart rate records from American crew members performing this countermeasure program show variations: for very light exercise levels the average heart rate is about 60% of maximal; for the more challenging programs there are peaks of near maximal heart rate during, for example, the treadmill sprints.

International Space Station (ISS)

During the assembly phase of the ISS three crew members will be traveling to and from the station on the Shuttle or on the Salyut vehicle, they will live and work on the station for 4–6 months. The assembly phase is expected to last about 5 yr and involve about 22 Shuttle flights and 41 Russian flights. After assembly has been completed, seven or eight crew members will spend approximate 4-mo periods on the station. The environmental guidelines for the ISS are: 76.5–79.4% N_2, 19.9–22.5% O_2, 0.7 to 1.0% CO_2, ambient temperature of 10–27°C (64.4–80.6°F), relative humidity of 25–70%, total pressure of 97.89–102.7 kPa (14.2–14.9 psi), and an intramodule air flow of 0.2 m·sec^{-1} (Wieland, 1998).

The exercise countermeasure program for the ISS will include at least 30 min of aerobic and 45 min of resistive exercise daily for 6 days each week, with the seventh day optional. The aerobic exercise will be performed on a treadmill or cycle on alternate days. The treadmill protocol involves continuous, moderate exercise at 70% of the maximal oxygen uptake ($\dot{V}O_{2\,max}$) and is designed to maintain aerobic endurance. The cycle protocol involves interval exercise with short bursts of intense exercise (90% $\dot{V}O_{2\,max}$) to maintain anaerobic as well as aerobic capacity. The resistance exercise devices are yet to be specified, but during initial ISS assembly they will include a pulley-type device to exercise specific upper and lower body muscle groups by repeated maximal contractions. The exercises will stress primarily postural and lower body muscle groups (e.g., squat, dead lift, heel raise). Initially, the resistive exercise device will be located in the first node of the ISS where environmental control may be limited. After assembly is completed and sufficient power is available, active resistive exercise devices providing concentric and eccentric exercise modalities will be available; they may then be located in a modular region of the station.

Extravehicular Activity

Because of the limited heat removal capacity of the EVA suit, the upper limit of energy utilization (body heat production) during EVA in the Gemini, Apollo, and Skylab flights was 225–300 kcal·hr^{-1} which corresponds to an oxygen uptake of 0.9–1.0 liters·min^{-1} (very light exercise). The average EVA time was about 6 and 4 hr for the Apollo and Skylab astronauts, respectively (Waligora and Horrigan, 1977). Vorobyev et al. (1986) reported similar mean energy expenditures (198–294 kcal·hr^{-1}) for two cosmonauts during 170–175 min of EVA; their average oxygen uptake was about 0.7 liters·min^{-1}.

The Shuttle EVA suit consists of a pressurized space suit and an integrated life-support system. The suit provides 4.3 psi pressure and a minimum oxygen concentration of 95%; it must protect crew members from the space vacuum and from ambient temperatures ranging from –118 to 136°C (–180.4 to 276.8°F). A liquid cooling garment within the EVA suit removes body heat by conduction; but cool air—4.4°C (39.9°F)—at the suit input port is recirculated throughout at a rate of about 2.83 liters·sec^{-1} to allow some evaporative heat loss. The combined cooling capacity of the suit is sufficient to evaporate sweat at work rates up to 400 kcal·hr^{-1} and will allow sustained work rates to 500 kcal·hr^{-1} without excessive thermal stress (Greenleaf, 1989a; Powell et al., 1994). This maximal rate of heat removal, equivalent to an oxygen uptake of about 1.7 liters·min^{-1}, is about 50% of the average maximal oxygen uptake of the astronaut corps, which is about 3.4 liters·min^{-1} or 45 ml·min^{-1}·kg^{-1} of body weight (Greenleaf, 1990). Constant exercise at a metabolic rate equivalent to 50% of peak VO_2 can be continued for 6–8 hr and will result in an equilibrium level of T_{co} of 38.0±0.1°C (100.4±0.2°F, Astrand, 1960), an optimal level for efficient work performance.

About 480 EVA's will be required during construction and maintenance of the ISS, and energy requirements will be similar to those of Shuttle EVA activities. Both American and Russian EVA suits will be employed. The Russian suit is inflated to a greater pressure (about 6 psi) and there is less thermal insulation, particularly for the hands. Cold injury to the hands has been a concern during American EVA's, but less so during Russian EVA's because they rely less on hand holds and use more free-tether techniques; for example, the Russians "stand down" during night cycles and tuck their gloved hands under the upper arms of the suit, whereas Americans tend to work throughout the dark cycles.

Postflight Egress and Reconditioning Program

A critical time for heat stress in crew members is during Shuttle entry and landing, particularly in the event of an emergency egress. Since the *Challenger* accident all crew members wear a launch and entry suit (LES) during launch, entry, and landing. This suit provides a counter-pressure system for limited protection against hypobaria, as well as thermal protection in case of immersion in cold water. However, the thermal properties of the suit, which were incorporated to protect against hypothermia, also create a potential risk for hyperthermia. This suit was provided with a cooling fan to shunt cabin air through the suit at a rate of 0.17 m^3·min^{-1}; this was apparently inadequate, however, because crew members frequently reported heat stress during flight. The ensuing enhanced vasodilation, high sweat rates, and dehydration probably contributed to the enhanced postflight orthostatic hypotension observed in some crew members (Bue et al., 1995). Indeed, with use of a heat strain model developed to predict heat casualties, Pandolf et al. (1995) entered the insulation values of the LES (1.29 clothing units when ventilated) and a predicted landing and emergency egress scenario postflight to calculate tolerance time for a crew member dehydrated by 3% body weight and after loss of heat acclimation. The scenario consisted of a 5.5 hr exposure to 24°C (75.2°F, 50% rh) at a low metabolic rate (100 kcal·hr^{-1}) to simulate normal pre-landing crew activities, followed by a 1.5 hr exposure to 35°C (95°F, 70% rh) at this same metabolic rate. Once the cooling supply to the suit was discontinued (simulating an emergency landing in which crew members would rush from the Shuttle), the tolerance time until T_{co} rose to the unacceptable level of 39°C (102.2°F) was only 6 min.

Starting with Shuttle flight STS-62 in 1994, crew members have worn a liquid cooling garment under the LES. This cooling garment weighs about 5 kg (11 lb); it consists of a thermoelectric system that chills water passing through tubes covering the surface of the body. The temperature of the system must be modulated manually by the crew member to maintain thermal comfort during entry and landing. In ground-based tests simulating entry, five subjects performed mild arm exercise (176 W) to simulate worst-case crew activities for 1.5 hr in a 32°C (89.6°F) environment. The liquid cooling-LES ensemble kept T_{co} from rising more than 0.5°C (0.9°F), and subjective ratings of thermal comfort began at "slightly warm" but were reduced to "neutral" and "comfortable" by the end of the session (Bue et al., 1995).

The LES-liquid cooling garment system is now worn by all crew members during Shuttle landings. Following a 16-day spaceflight, intestinal temperatures of four of the crew were monitored during landing while they wore the LES system and compared with those obtained at the same time of day, 48 hr earlier (Rimmer et al., 1999). Intestinal temperature was elevated significantly by about 0.3–0.5°C (0.5–0.9°F) during the pre-deorbit preparation and landing, suggesting that the cooling capacity of the LES system is inadequate to handle body heat loads during nominal landing. This leads to further concern about the outcome of a true emergency situation in which crew metabolic rate and heat production could be much higher. Recently, Bishop et al. (1999) measured metabolic rate during the ambulation phase of a simulated egress; metabolic rates varied between 600 kcal·hr^{-1} without G-suit inflation to almost 800 kcal·hr^{-1} with the G-suit inflated maximally to 1.5 psi.

Lunar/Mars Exploration

Lunar/Mars expeditions would expose crew members to extended periods of reduced gravity: microgravity in the spaceship and partial Earth gravity while living and working on the surface. These environmental conditions will require more sophisticated life-support systems than are presently available.

Moon

The dominant features of a lunar stay are the near vacuum environment and great extremes of ambient temperature. The primary constituents of the lunar atmosphere are neon-20, helium, hydrogen, and argon-40. The length of the lunar day is approximately 15 Earth days, which enables the temperature at the lunar surface at the mid-equatorial region to reach 121°C (249.8°F) during the day and –122°C (–187.6°F) at night. Much lower temperatures to –198°C (–324.4°F) occur in the more shaded polar regions (Horton, 1997). Twelve Apollo crew members spent a total of 160 hr on the lunar surface at one-sixth of Earth's gravity. Metabolic rates during the astronauts' average 6-hr extravehicular activities were $225-300$ kcal·hr^{-1}, and their activity may have been restricted owing to the limited cooling capacity of their EVA suits (Greenleaf, 1989a).

Mars

Mars has a much more complicated environment than that of the Moon; for example, it has an extremely thin atmosphere, that results in meteorological phenomena similar to those on Earth. The eccentricity of Mars' orbit results in large variations in its distance from the Sun, and those variations produce distinct seasons. The Martian day is about 37 min longer than Earth's. Mars atmosphere is different from that of Earth in that it consists mostly of CO_2 (95.3%) with small amounts of N_2 (2.7%), Ar (1.6%), O_2 (0.13%), CO (0.07%), and water vapor (0.03%). The atmospheric pressure on Mars varies (with the seasons) between 7.0 and 10.0 millibars, a result of sublimation of CO_2 in the polar ice caps. The atmosphere on Mars makes transfer of heat possible through convection which can be accelerated by winds which reach speeds in excess of 20 m·sec^{-1} (45 mph) during dust storms. The average temperature on the planet surface varies from –98°C (–144.4°F) to –2°C (28.4°F), with diurnal variations of as great as 62°C (111.6°F) or as little as 13°C (23.4°F) depending on the season and location. In southern regions summer surface temperatures can reach an Earth-like 20°C (68°F). One Martian scenario has crew members traveling for approximately 1 year in weightlessness to reach the planet, then spending up to 3 years on the surface at about 0.38 Earth's gravity before embarking on the 1-year return trip, also in weightlessness. Intense exercise, pharmacological countermeasures, or both would be necessary to prevent life-threatening changes in muscle and bone mass during extended stays in such reduced gravity environments.

SPACEFLIGHT THERMOREGULATION

Maintenance of a constant T_{co} is dependent on maintaining an appropriate balance between factors that increase body temperature (metabolism) and those that reduce it (heat-loss responses). In humans resting in a temperate environment the primary avenue of heat loss is through nonevaporative mechanisms: radiation, conduction, and convection. The most important is convective loss from the skin to the environment which accounts for roughly 75% of the total body heat loss (Robinson, 1949). During exercise in a hot environment, evaporation becomes the primary avenue for heat loss in humans. Sweat that does not evaporate, but drips from the skin, does not produce body cooling. There are no direct data regarding the effects of weightlessness on total heat balance in humans.

Heat Production

Energy expenditure during spaceflight is probably similar to that on Earth (Lane et al., 1997). The caloric deficit reported in some crew members, especially early in a mission, likely resulted from a decrease in food (caloric) intake rather than from an increased energy output.

Heat production during exercise could be altered if there were a change in mechanical efficiency. Mechanical efficiency was estimated during Skylab missions from measurements of oxygen consumption during exercise at 150 W. Six of the nine Skylab crew had a small but statistically significant increase in mechanical efficiency during cycle-ergometer exercise in flight (Michel et al., 1977). This increase may have been related to the increased fitness of these particular Skylab crew members rather than to a true change in metabolic efficiency caused by weightlessness.

Heat Loss

The two primary avenues of body heat loss that may be affected by spaceflight are convection and evaporation. Convective heat loss depends on the nature and rate of flow of air across the surface of the skin (the surface area for heat exchange), and the temperature gradient between the skin and the surrounding air (Hardy, 1949). At very low air flows (less than 0.12 m·sec^{-1}), body heat loss occurs primarily by natural convection in which heat exchange occurs when the air nearest the skin surface becomes warmer and lighter than the surrounding air. In a 1-G environment this warm air rises from the skin, thereby removing body heat. In flight, the warm air would not rise and this lack of free convection could lead to increasing heat buildup. Novak et al. (1980) confirmed that, at air flows of less than 2 m·sec^{-1}, there was an impairment in convective heat loss from an artificially heated metal cylinder in flight. At air flows greater than 2 m·sec^{-1} the turbulent flow and forced convective heat loss drastically increased heat loss to levels similar to those in a 1-G environment. These findings may be further complicated in humans where clothing may impede the effect of air flow for enhancing convection.

Skin temperature is a critical determinant of convective heat loss in humans because heat is transferred to the surface of the skin by the circulating blood. Tizil (1974) reported lower resting skin temperatures and hypo-reactive vasomotor responses to thermal stress during 12 days of bed rest (BR), and others have suggested that there is reduced skin blood flow during exercise (Greenleaf and

Reese, 1980; Lee et al., 1999) or heat exposure (Crandall et al., 1994) after BR. Thus, the lack of natural convection and a delay in transfer of heat to the skin surface could significantly impair convective heat loss in weightlessness.

The effect of spaceflight on evaporative heat loss is unclear. Lack of the effect of gravity would result in formation of a sheet of sweat on the skin surface; since evaporative heat loss is dependent on the wetted surface area, this sheet should increase evaporative heat loss. However, this layer of sweat on the skin must evaporate to release body heat. Formation of such a thick layer of water on the skin may create a situation in which skin temperature is insufficient to raise the skin's surface water to the critical temperature necessary for evaporation (Hardy, 1949). Also, excessive skin wetting could inhibit sweating by blocking the orifices of the sweat glands. Thus, both impaired transfer of heat to the skin because of altered vasomotor regulation and an increased volume of surface water resulting from less drippage may impede evaporative heat loss. This would greatly affect exercise thermal tolerance when evaporation is the primary avenue for heat loss.

Circadian Shifts

The circadian effect of body T_{co} is markedly altered during spaceflight (Lhagwa, 1984). Crew members on spacecraft orbiting Earth experience complete day/night cycles approximately every 90 min. This change in light cycling has been postulated to produce changes in the secretion of brain neurotransmitters, such as melatonin and growth hormone, which may be responsible for disruption of sleep patterns and of the normal 24-hr oscillations in T_{co}. Sleep patterns may also be disturbed by other effects during flight such as prolonged working days, noise, and phase shifting of sleep periods which may in turn reduce the circadian changes in T_{co}. The outcome of circadian desynchronization may be fatigue and a "sluggish" response to thermal stressors (Krupina and Tizul, 1977). During intraplanetary missions this light/dark cycle may completely disappear until landing on the surface when a new circadian cycle may be induced.

Deconditioning/Deacclimation

Most American astronauts are moderately fit; their average aerobic exercise capacity ($\dot{V}O_{2\,max}$) is about 45 ml·kg^{-1}·min^{-1}. They live and work in and around Houston, Texas, a warm, humid area in which they have probably acquired some degree of heat acclimatization to the ambient environment. Both Shuttle and ISS ambient conditions are temperate (see above) so, unless the crew maintains a rigorous in-flight exercise regimen, they will most likely experience some loss of this acclimatization and a decrease in aerobic conditioning. Both deconditioning (Greenleaf and Reese, 1980) and deacclimation (Roberts et al., 1977) compromise thermoregulatory function. With a loss of aerobic capacity, there is decoupling in both sweating and skin blood flow responses to a rise in core temperature resulting in a faster rise in body temperature during exercise. With loss of heat acclimation

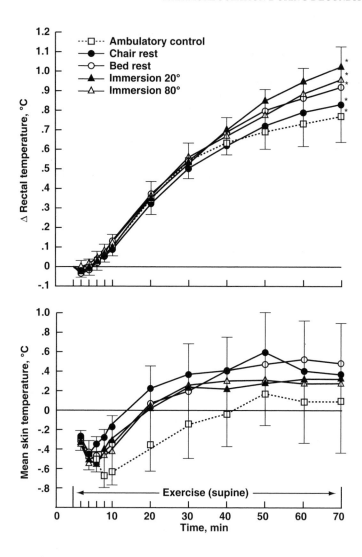

Figure 10.1 Changes in rectal temperature and mean skin temperature during exercise after chair rest, bed rest, and immersion. (From Greenleaf et al., 1996, with permission.)

there is delay in onset of sweating and vasodilation, again resulting in a greater body heat storage before heat loss responses are activated (Roberts et al., 1977). These two effects are additive resulting in a greater potential for heat exhaustion and fatigue when they occur simultaneously.

The goal on ISS missions will be to maintain ground-level aerobic capacity and each crew member will spend approximately 90 min·day^{-1} performing exercises which should be sufficient to maintain aerobic fitness. Maintenance of aerobic capacity should help preserve thermoregulatory responses during exercise in a cool environment, but it may not be protective in a warmer environment or under conditions of uncompensable heat loss such as when wearing the LES or the EVA suit with insufficient cooling.

Addition of an orthostatic stress immediately postflight may compromise exercise and thermal responses, even for crew members who have maintained aerobic fitness. Even though the aerobic capacity of three crew members was maintained during the Skylab 3 and 4 missions (Sawin et al., 1975), when subjected to 1-G on landing they experienced significant reduction in aerobic capacity (Michel et al., 1977).

Hypovolemia

One well-known effect of spaceflight is a decrease in blood volume (hypovolemia). Both plasma volume (PV) and red cell mass are reduced during the first 30–60 days of a mission before reaching equilibrium (Fortney et al., 1996). Some data suggest increases in either the interstitial (Greenleaf, 1989b) or cellular fluid compartments (Leach et al., 1996) to compensate for the reduction in blood volume; total body water (TBW) has been reported to be unchanged during relatively short-duration (14–16-day) Shuttle missions despite significant reduction in the extracellular fluid volume (ECV, Leach et al., 1996).

A loss of blood volume on Earth of the magnitude occurring during spaceflight results in impaired sweating and skin blood flow (Nadel et al., 1980; Fortney at al., 1981). In space, however, the effects of hypohydration on thermoregulatory responses may differ in that reduction of blood volume is probably an appropriate adaptation in humans without vascular hydrostatic gradients. The central blood volume of a resting astronaut is increased transiently during the first 4–6 days of flight and then returns toward the preflight level (Charles and Lathers, 1991). However, when the peripheral blood vessels dilate, thereby shunting blood away from the core to the skin surface during exercise, the smaller central blood volume may cause unloading of cardiopulmonary baroreflexes which would attenuate the degree of peripheral vasodilation leading to faster heat storage. Similarly, during profuse sweating with a smaller blood volume in flight, plasma osmolality could increase at a faster rate thus initiating fluid-conserving responses which may reduce body sweating and also result in greater heat storage.

BED-REST THERMOREGULATION

Data from short-term (<24 hr) head-down tilt (HDT) or more prolonged BR studies indicate no significant change in basal or resting body T_{co} (Fortney 1987; Greenleaf, 1989a). But there is a significant "excessive" increase in T_{co} during controlled isotonic or isometric exercise regimens after BR-deconditioning, which indicates altered thermoregulatory mechanisms. These altered mechanisms occur in both women (Fortney, 1987) and men (Greenleaf and Reese, 1980). From these exercise studies and from passive heating studies (Crandall et al., 1994), the major conclusion is that reduced vascular conductance (mainly peripheral blood flow) was responsible for attenuating body heat dissipation and thus causing an increase in T_{co}; that is, the cause was mainly a peripheral rather than a central-acting mechanism. Apparently, decreased sweating does not play a major role even in the presence of reduced PV, which can reduce sweating in ambulatory subjects (Greenleaf and Castle, 1971). Chronically decreased TBW and ECV (including PV) during prolonged BR is a major function of the adaptive syndrome such that the subjects can no longer be considered hypohydrated and hypovolemic; that is, they are euhydrated with chronically reduced TBW and ECV. Therefore, the hypovolemia during BR may no longer be a feasible physiological stimulus for the excessive hyperthermia as long as the subjects remain in the horizontal or head-down (anti-hydrostatic) positions.

Even though Mack et al. (1994) concluded that active cutaneous vasodilation in ambulatory subjects was dependent on interaction between supine exercise intensity and PV, Greenhaff and Clough (1989) reported that $\dot{V}O_{2\,max}$, and not heart rate, mean skin temperature (T_{sk}), or rectal temperature (T_{re}), was the most important predictor of exercise sweating rate. The effect of hypovolemia in reducing sweating and peripheral blood flow has not been studied satisfactorily in deconditioned subjects (see spaceflight results below).

Thermoregulation during supine submaximal exercise (51% $\dot{V}O_{2\,max}$) in hydrated men with no additional hydration can be altered after only 6 hr of chair rest (CR) or BR, or water immersion (WI) at body angles of 20° and 80° (Greenleaf et al., 1996). The post-conditioning hierarchy of the ΔT_{re} at 70 min of exercise was approximately related to the severity of the treatments (Figure 10.1, upper panel): the WI responses were greatest (ΔT_{re}: at 20° = 1.03±0.09°C (1.86±0.16 °F); at 80° = 0.96±0.13°C (1.73±0.23 °F); then BR (ΔT_{re} = 0.92±0.13 °C) (1.66±0.23 °F); CR (ΔT_{re} = 0.83±0.08°C) (1.43±0.14 °F); and finally, ambulatory control (ΔT_{re} = 0.77±0.13°C) (1.39±0.23 °F). Those ΔT_{re} curves were not different from each other during the first 30 min of exercise further emphasizing the importance of the heat dissipation mechanisms, which do not appear to be fully activated. Factors that had essentially no effect on the T_{re} were limb (arm, calf) sweating and arm skin or total blood flow. Factors moderately correlated with T_{re} were total body sweating ($r = 0.60$), skin conductance ($r = 0.57$), and mean skin temperature ($r = 0.49$, Figure 10.1, lower panel).

From these and other findings (Fortney et al., 1996; Greenleaf et al., 1982; Kollias et al., 1976; Luu et al., 1990) it would seem that multiple factors (mechanisms) are involved in deconditioning-induced exercise excessive hyperthermia. These include interaction between attenuation of heat transfer from mainly working muscles to the skin, as well as reduced evaporative heat loss. Perhaps more emphasis should be placed on the variability of cerebral blood flow, as well as on the function of central thermo- and osmo-receptors (Kozlowski et al., 1980). These factors may play a greater role in response to the 700-ml cephalic fluid shift (Arborelius et al., 1972) that takes place in these deconditioning procedures, especially in the WI studies during which greater exercise ΔT_{re} occurred.

THERMOREGULATION DURING THERMONEUTRAL IMMERSION

Rectal temperature remains within a range of 0.2°C (36.7–36.9°C) (98.1–98.4°F) during 8 hr of WI to the neck at the thermoneutral water temperature of 34.4°C (93.9°F) (Greenleaf et al., 1980, Figure 10.2). Boutelier, Timbal, and Colin (1973) also reported that T_{re} remained constant within 0.1°C (36.7–36.8°C) (98.1–98.2°F) during 2 hr of WI at 33–34°C (91.4–93.2°F); they also observed a slight drop in T_{re} within the first 2 hr at a water temperature just below 35°C (95°F). Craig and Dvorak (1966) recommended that the optimal thermoneutral water temperature range was 35.0–35.5°C (95.0–95.9°F).

Mean skin temperature in non-obese subjects remains within ±1°C (±1.8°F) of the water temperature, although local T_{sk} may exhibit greater variability. Moderate variations in body-fat content do not affect body thermal conductivity because peripheral arterial circulation short circuits subcutaneous fat on its way to feed the dermal arteriolar plexuses (Boutleier et al., 1973). Body thermal conductivity in thermoneutral water is essentially the same as in 22.5°C (72.5°F) air where similar T_{re} levels (Figure 10.2) are a result of the similar body thermal conductivities, as well as the thermal conductivity of water which is greater than that of air.

As mentioned above, the change and final level of T_{re} during supine leg cycle ergometer exercise (51% $\dot{V}O_{2\,max}$) after WI of 1.03±0.09°C and 37.96±0.12°C (20° angle); and 0.96±0.13°C and 37.90±0.18 °C (80° angle), respectively, were similar to those from a prior study (Greenleaf et al., 1985). This latter study was conducted supine with leg exercise at 50% $\dot{V}O_{2\,max}$ where the respective change and final T_{re} were 1.1 and 38.1°C (air control), and 0.9 and 38.3°C after WI (Figure 10.3). Neither study showed any significant differences in calculated skin heat conductance data between the control and experimental treatments; reduced sweating (evaporative heat loss) could not account for the higher exercise T_{re} in air after water immersion.

The mechanism for the exercise excessive hyperthermia in air after BR (Fortney, 1987; Greenleaf and Reese, 1980) and spaceflight (Fortney et al., 1998) appears to be reduced heat conductance from the body core (active muscles) to the periphery because of decreased peripheral blood flow. Most data indicate little or no effect of thermoneutral WI or moderate submaximal exercise on airway closure (Derion et al., 1992) or on cardiorespiratory response in air at a dry-bulb temperature (T_{db}) of 22°C (71.6°F) such as respiratory gas exchange, end-tidal gas tensions, alveolar ventilation, respiratory frequency, cardiac output, or pulse rate (Denison et al., 1972). However, total body or head-out WI generally causes reduced forearm and calf blood flow with accompanying increase in vascular resistance (vaso-constriction) followed by hyperemia in air after emerging from the water (Campbell et al., 1969). On the other hand, Echt et al. 1974) observed reduced venous tone (vasodilation) in the forearm during prolonged (3-hr) head-out WI. This vasodilation, if uncompensated, would facilitate increased heat loss during exercise in air, but that does not appear to be the case. Perhaps there is a compensatory post-immersion, exercise-induced peripheral vasoconstriction that contributes to the

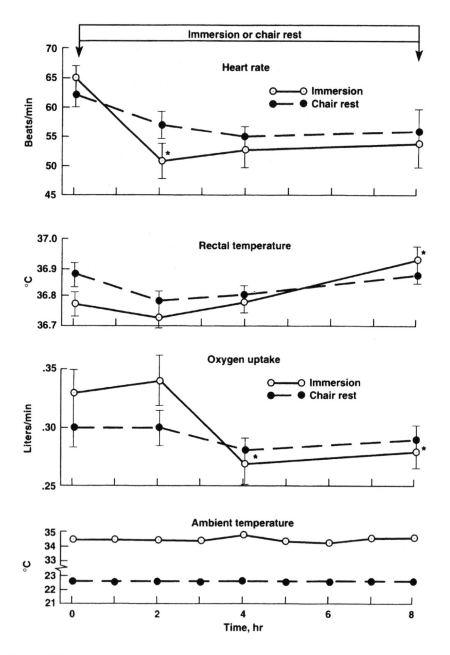

Figure 10.2 Comparison of changes in heart rate, rectal temperature, and oxygen uptake during immersion or chair rest. (From Greenleaf et al., 1980, with permission.)

excessive hyperthermia. Thus, there is no clear primary mechanism for the generally higher exercise core temperature after short-term immersion deconditioning.

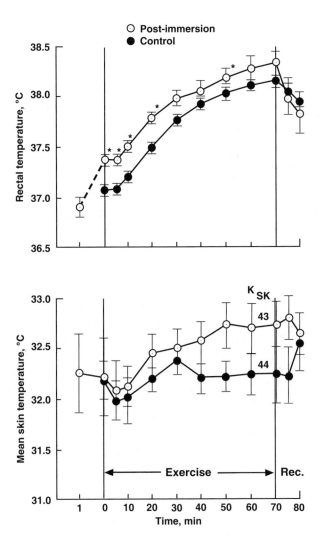

Figure 10.3 Rectal temperature and mean skin temperature responses to exercise following control and immersion conditions. K_{sk} = calculated skin heat conductance. (From Greenleaf et al., 1985, with permission.)

SPACEFLIGHT EXERCISE THERMOREGULATION

There are no direct measurements of heat balance during exercise in spaceflight. However, submaximal exercise and thermoregulatory responses of two crew members during a 115-day Shuttle–Mir mission were studied preflight and at 5 days postflight (Fortney et al., 1998). Both crew members were able to complete a supine

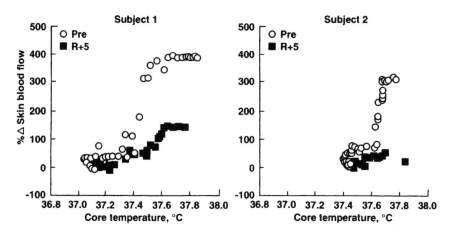

Figure 10.4   Skin blood flow responses in two crew members after 115 days of spaceflight. (From Fortney et al., 1998, with permission.)

exercise protocol (20 min at 40% $\dot{V}O_{2\,max}$ and 20 min at 65% $\dot{V}O_{2\,max}$) preflight with minimal stress and with heart rates of only 123 and 137 bpm. Postflight, however, the exercise was discontinued after 8–9 min into the 65% $\dot{V}O_{2\,max}$ work level when both crew members began having difficulty maintaining the pedaling frequency and complained of leg fatigue. The exercise was terminated when the heart rate exceeded the highest value from the preflight test. The body T_{co} of each crew member after exercise had been stopped approached the final preflight temperature. Since resting T_{co} were similar and the total exercise time was approximately 35% shorter postflight, the rate of rise of T_{co} was greater postflight. From these and previous BR data (Lee et al., 1999), it appears that heat production was not altered; and thus, the primary reason for the greater rate of rise in T_{co} was impaired heat loss from altered vasodilatory (Figure 10.4) and sweating (Figure 10.5) responses.

For any given T_{co} during exercise after flight, the skin blood flow and sweating responses are greatly reduced resulting in faster and greater body heat storage; thus, if exercise were to be continued there would be a greater probability of heat injury.

CLINICAL APPLICATIONS

Many of the findings discussed above may have direct application for people on Earth. For example, in an attempt to reduce heat strain in astronauts wearing protective clothing, special cooling garments and temperature-monitoring equipment have been and continue to be developed. The cooling garment worn underneath the EVA suit is being evaluated for use in firefighter's ensembles by incorporating many of the cooling properties of the suit to increase their thermal tolerance from the

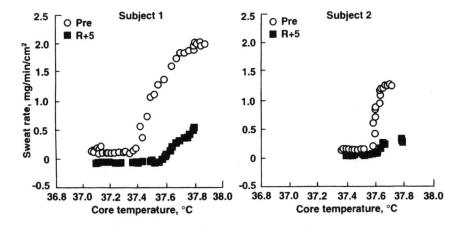

Figure 10.5 Sweat rate responses in two crew members after 115 days of spaceflight. (From Fortney et al., 1998, with permission.)

present 10–20 min to at least 1 hr. The isolated environment provided by the EVA suit has also been used for the management of immunodeficient patients, such as the well publicized "Bubble Boy" (Guerra and Shearer, 1986). A suit with UV protection has been used by children with xeroderma pigmentosum, a rare disease in which sunlight can be life threatening. The cooling system from the EVA suit has also been used in developing garments for patients with multiple sclerosis, spina bifida, cerebral palsy, and other disorders.

Non-rectal temperature sensors used for monitoring core temperature in crew members have been evaluated. The rectal probe produces much more discomfort in flight than before flight. This discomfort induced development of ingestible telemetry pill systems (Human Technologies Inc., St. Petersburg, FL; Personal Electronic, Inc., Wellesley, MA). These pills and monitors could provide continuous accurate readings of T_{co} during cardiac transplant surgeries or hyperthermic treatment of cancer patients, for circadian monitoring of patients with endocrine disorders, during rehabilitation of prolonged BR patients, or when reconditioning athletes who suddenly resume training in a hot climate.

Thermoregulatory studies conducted in weightlessness offer a unique opportunity to study basic physiological processes. For example, the unusual combi- nation of a reduced extracellular fluid volume without significant change in total body water may provide new insight into the role of extravascular volume receptors for control of cardiovascular and thermal reflex responses. The changes in autonomic reflexes which result from the altered blood flow distribution may mimic changes that occur with aging or in certain disease states (idiopathic hypotension). Finally, an understanding of the susceptibility to heat injuries that can occur under conditions of only moderately elevated body core temperatures, and the use of cooling garments to prevent such injuries, may have occupational or military applications for workers who perform in environments where impermeable clothing is worn for extended periods.

REFERENCES

Arborelius, Jr., M., Balldin, U. I., Lilja, B., Lundgren, C. E. G. (1972) Hemodynamic changes in man during immersion with the head above water. *Aerospace Med.* **43**: 592–598.

Astrand, I. (1960) Aerobic work capacity in men and women with special reference to age. *Acta Physiol. Scand.* **49**: *Suppl* **169**: 1–92.

Bishop, P. A., Lee, S. M. C., Conza, N. E., Clapp, L. L., Moore, A. D., Williams, W. J., Guilliams, M. E., Greenisen, M.C. (1999) Carbon dioxide accumulation, walking performance, and metabolic cost in the NASA Launch and Entry Suit. *Aviat. Space Environ. Med.* **70**: 656–665.

Boutelier, C., Timbal, J., Colin, J. (1973) Conductance thermique du corps humain en immersion a la neutralite thermique et en amibance froide. *Arch. Sci. Physiol.* **27**: 189–205 (NASA technical translation F-16258).

Bue, G. C., Conger, B. C., Hooper, P. E., Chang, C., Sauser, B. (1995) Shuttle launch entry suit liquid cooling system thermal performance. 25th Conference on Environmental Systems, SAE Technical Paper Series 951546.

Campbell, L. B., Gooden, B. A., Lehman, R. G., Pym, J. (1969) Simultaneous calf and forearm blood flow during immersion in man. *Aust. J. Exp. Med. Sci.* **47**: 747–754.

Charles, J. B., Lathers, C. M. (1991) Cardiovascular adaptations to spaceflight. *J. Clin. Pharmacol.* **31**: 1010–1023.

Convertino, V. A., Greenleaf, J. E., Bernauer, E. M. (1980) Role of thermal and exercise factors in the mechanism of hypervolemia. *J. Appl. Physiol.* **48**: 657–664.

Craig, A. B., Jr., Dvorak, M. (1966) Thermal regulation during water immersion. *J. Appl. Physiol.* **21**: 1577–1585.

Crandall, C. G., Johnson, J. M., Convertino, V. A., Raven, R. B., Engelke, K.A. (1994) Altered thermoregulatory responses after 15 days of head-down tilt. *J. Appl. Physiol.* **77**: 1863–1867.

Czeisler, C. A., Chiasera, A. J., Duffy, J. F. (1991) Research on sleep, circadian rhythms and aging: applications to manned spaceflight. *Exp. Gerontol.* **26**: 217–232.

Denison, D. M., Wagner, D., Kingaby, G. L., West, J. B. (1972) Cardiorespiratory responses to exercise in air and under water. *J. Appl. Physiol.* **33**: 426–430.

Derion, T., Guy, H. J. B., Tsukimoto, K., Schaffartzik, W., Prediletto, R., Poole, D. C., Knight, D. R., Wagner, P.D. (1992) Ventilation–perfusion relationships in the lung during head-out water immersion. *J. Appl. Physiol.* **72**: 64–72.

Echt, M., Lange, L., Gauer, O. H. (1974) Changes in peripheral venous tone and central transmural venous pressure during immersion in a thermo-neutral bath. *Pflügers Arch.* **352**: 211–217.

Fortney, S. M. (1987) Thermoregulatory Adaptations to Inactivity. In *Adaptive Physiology to Stressful Environments*, edited by S. Samueloff and M.K. Yousef, CRC Press, Boca Raton, FL, pp. 75–83.

Fortney, S. M., Mikhaylov, V., Lee, S. M. C., Kobzev,Y., Gonzalez, R., and Greenleaf, J. E. (1998) Body temperature and thermoregulation during submaximal exercise after 115-day spaceflight. *Aviat. Space Environ. Med.* **69**: 137–141.

Fortney, S. M., Nadel, E. R., Wenger, C. B., and Bove, J. R. (1981) Effect of blood volume on sweating rate and body fluids in exercising humans. *J. Appl. Physiol.* **51**: 1594–1600.

Fortney, S. M., Schneider, V. S., and Greenleaf, J. E. (1996) The physiology of bed rest. In *Handbook of Physiology, Section 4, Environmental Physiology*, edited by M.J. Fregley and C. M. Blatteis. Oxford University Press: New York, Vol. 2, Chap. 39, pp. 889–939.

Greenhaff, P. L., and Clough, P. J. (1989) Predictors of sweat loss in man during prolonged exercise. *Eur. J. Appl. Physiol.* **58**: 348–352.

Greenleaf, J. E. (1989a) Energy and thermal regulation during bed rest and spaceflight. *J. Appl. Physiol.* **67**: 507–516.

Greenleaf, J. E. (1989b) Hormonal regulation of fluid and electrolytes during prolonged bed rest: implications for microgravity. In *Hormonal Regulation of Fluid and Electrolytes*, edited by J. R. Claybaugh and C. E. Wade, Plenum Publ. Corp., New York, pp. 216–232.

Greenleaf, J. E. (1990) Human exercise capabilities in space. 20th Intersociety Conference on Environmental Systems, SAE Technical Paper 901200, 11 pp.

Greenleaf, J. E., and Castle, B. L. (1971) Exercise temperature regulation in man during hypohydration and hyperhydration. *J. Appl. Physiol.* **30**: 847–853.

Greenleaf, J. E., Hutchinson, T., Shaffer-Bailey, M., and Looft-Wilson, R. (1996) Exercise thermoregulation after 6 hr chair rest, 6° head-down bed-rest, and water immersion deconditioning in men. *Eur. J. Appl. Physiol.* **72**: 303–309.

Greenleaf, J. E., and Reese, R. D. (1980) Exercise thermoregulation after 14 days of bed rest. *J. Appl. Physiol.* **48**: 72–78.

Greenleaf, J. E,, Shvartz, E., Kravik, S., and Keil, L.C. (1980) Fluid shifts and endocrine responses during chair rest and water immersion in man. *J. Appl. Physiol.* **48**: 79–88.

Greenleaf, J. E., Silverstein, L., Bliss, J., Langenheim, V., Rossow, H., and Chao, C. (1982) Physiological responses to prolonged bed rest and fluid immersion in man: A compendium of research (1974–1980). Moffett Field, CA, NASA TM-81324, 110 pp.

Greenleaf, J. E., Spaul, W. A., Kravik, S. E., Wong, N., and Elder, C. A. (1985) Exercise thermoregulation in men after 6 hours of immersion. *Aviat. Space Environ. Med.* **56**: 15–18.

Guerra, I. C., and Shearer, W. T. (1986) Environmental control in management of immunodeficient patients: experience with "David." *Clin. Immunol. Immunopathol.* **40**: 128–135.

Hardy, J. D. (1949) Heat Transfer. *In Physiology of Heat Regulation*, edited by L.H. Newburgh, W.B. Saunders, Co.: Philadelphia, PA, pp. 78–108.

Horton, R. D. (1997) Thermal environment evaluation of EVA on the Moon and Mars. Houston, TX, Lockheed Martin Tech. Memo. LMSSS 32509.

Kollias, J., Van Derveer, D., Dorchak, K. J., and Greenleaf, J. E. (1976) Physiologic responses to water immersion in man: A compendium of research. Washington, DC, NASA TM X-3308, 87 pp.

Kozlowski, S., Greenleaf, J. E., Turlejska, E., and Nazar, K. (1980) Extracellular hyperomolality and body temperature during physical exercise in dogs. *Am. J. Physiol. Regulatory Integrative Comp. Physiol.* **239**: R180–R183.

Krupina, T. N., and Tizul, A. Ya. (1977) Clinical aspects of changes in the nervous system in the course of 49-day antiorthostatic hypokinesia. *Kosm. Biol. Aviakosm. Med.* **11**: 26–31.

Lane, H. W., Gretebeck, R. J., Schoeller, D. A., Davis-Street, J., Socki, R. A., and Gibson, E. K. (1997) Comparison of ground-based and spaceflight energy expenditure and water turnover in middle-aged healthy male U.S. astronauts. *Am. J. Clin. Nutr.* **65**: 4–12.

Leach, C. S., Alfrey, C. P., Suki, W. N., Leonard, J. I., Rambaut, P. C., Inners, L. D., Smith, S. M., Lane, H. W., and Krauhs, J. M. (1996) Regulation of body fluid compartments during short-term spaceflight. *J. Appl. Physiol.* **81**: 105–116.

Leach, C. S., Leonard, J. I., Rambaut, P. C, and Johnson, P.C. (1978) Evaporative water loss in man in a gravity-free envionment. *J. Appl. Physiol.* **45**: 430–436.

Lee, S. M. C., Williams, W. J., and Schneider, S. M. (2002) Role of skin blood flow and sweating rate in exercise thermoregulation after bed rest. *J. Appl. Physiol.* **92**: 2026–2034.

Leithead, C. S., and Lind, A. R. (1964) *Heat Stress and Heat Disorders*. F.A. Davis Co.: Philadelphia, PA, pp. 195–196.

Lhagwa, L. (1984) Circadian rhythm of human body temperature during spaceflights. *Kosm. Biol. Aviakosm. Med.* **13**: 15–18.

Luu, P. B., Ortiz, V., Barnes, P. R, and Greenleaf, J. E. (1990) Physiological responses to prolonged bed rest in humans: A compendium of research (1981–1988). Moffett Field, CA, NASA TM-102249, 134 pp.

Mack, G. W., Nose, H., Takamata, A., Okuno, T., and Morimoto, T. (1994) Influence of exercise intensity and plasma volume on active cutaneous vasodilation in humans. *Med. Sci. Sports Exerc.* **26**: 209–216.

Michel, E. L., Rummel, J. A., Sawin, C. F., Buderer, M. C., and Lem, J. D. (1977) Results of Skylab medical experiment M171-metabolic activity. In *Biomedical Results of Skylab*, edited by R. S. Johnson and L. F. Dietlein, Washington, DC, NASA SP-377, pp. 372–387.

Nadel, E. R., Fortney, S. M., and Wenger, C. B. (1980) Effect of hydration state on circulatory and thermal regulations. *J. Appl. Physiol.* **49**: 715–721.

Novak, L., Prokopova, L., Genin, A. M., and Golov, V. K. (1980) Results of "heat transfer 1" experiment conducted aboard the Cosmos-936 biosatellite. *Kosm. Biol. Aviakosm. Med.* **14**: 73–76.

O'Brien, C., Young, A. J., and Sawka, M. N. (1998) Hypohydration and thermoregulation in cold air. *J. Appl. Physiol.* **84**: 185–189.

Pandolf, K. B., Stroschein, L. A., Gonzalez, R. R., and Sawka, M. N. (1995) Predicting human heat strain and performance with application to space operations. *Aviat. Space Environ. Med.* **66**: 364–368.

Powell, M. R., Horrigan, Jr., D. J., Waligora, J. M., and Norfleet, W. T. (1994) Extravehicular activities. In *Space Biology and Medicine*, edited by A. E. Nicogossian, C. L. Huntoon, and S. L. Pool, Lea and Febiger: Philadelphia, PA, pp. 128–140.

Pugh, L. G. C. E., Corbett, J. L., and Johnson, R. H. (1967) Rectal temperatures, weight losses, and sweat rates in marathon running. *J. Appl. Physiol.* **23**: 347–352.

Putcha, L., Berens, K. L., Marshburn, T. H., Ortega, H. J., and Billica, R. D. (1999) Pharmaceutical use by U.S. astronauts on Space Shuttle missions. *Aviat. Space Environ. Med.* **70**: 705–708.

Rimmer, D. W., Dijk, D-J., Ronda, J. M., Hoyt, R., and Pawelczyk, J. A. (1999) Efficiency of liquid cooling garments to minimize heat strain during space shuttle deorbit and landing. *Med. Sci. Sports Exerc.* **31**: S305.

Roberts, M. F., Wenger, C. B., Stolwijk, J. A. J, and Nadel, E. R. (1977) Skin blood flow and sweating changes following exercise training and heat acclimation. *J. Appl. Physiol.* **43**: 133–137.

Robinson, S. (1949) Physiological adjustments to heat. In *Physiology of Heat Regulation*, edited by L. H. Newburgh, W. B. Saunders, Co.: Philadelphia, PA, pp. 193–231.

Robinson, S. (1963) Temperature regulation in exercise. *Pediatrics* **32**: (part II): 691–702.

Sawin, C. F., Rummel, J. A., and Michel, E. L. Instrumented personal exercise during long-duration space flights. *Aviat. Space Environ. Med.* **46**: 394–400.

Sawka , M. N., Young, A. J., Latzka, W. A., Neufer, P. D., Quigley, M. D., and Pandolf, K. B. (1992) Human tolerance to heat strain during exercise: influence of hydration. *J. Appl. Physiol.* **73**: 368–375.

Shibolet, S., Lancaster, M. C., and Danon, Y. (1976) Heat stroke: A review. *Aviat. Space Environ. Med.* **47**: 280–301.

Smith, D. J. (1980) Protective clothing and thermal stress. *Ann. Occup. Hyg.* **23**: 217–224.

Tanaka, M., Brisson, G. R., and Volle, M. A. (1978) Body temperatures in relation to heart rate for workers wearing impermeable clothing in a hot environment. *Am. Indust. Hyg. Assoc. J.* **39**: 885–890.

Tizul, A.Ya. (1973) The function of thermoregulation in protracted limitation of motor activity (hypokinesia). *Z. Nevropatol. Psikhiat.* **73**: 1791–1794, (NASA TT F-15,566, 1974).

Vorobyev, Y. I., Gazenko, O. G., Shulzhenko, Y. B., Grigoryev, A. I., Barer, A. S., Yegorov, A. D., and Skiba, I. A. (1986) Preliminary results of medical investigation during 5-month spaceflight aboard Slayut 7-Soyuz-T complex. *Kosm. Biol. Aviakosm. Med.* **20**: 27–34.

Waligora, J. M., and Horrigan, Jr., D. J. (1977) Metabolic cost of extravehicular activities. In *Biomedical Results from Skylab*, edited by R.S. Johnson and L.F. Dietlein, Washington, DC, NASA SP-377, pp. 395–399.

Waligora, J. M., Powell, M. R., and Sauer, R. L. (1994) Spacecraft life support systems. In *Space Physiology and Medicine*, edited by A. E. Nicogossian, C.L. Huntoon, and S.L. Pool, Lea and Febiger: Philadelphia, PA, pp. 109–127.

Wieland, P. O. (1998) Living together in space: the design and operation of the life support systems on the International Space Station. Washington, DC, NASA TM-206956, vol. 1.

Subject Index